What Others Are Saying About This Book

"Debbie and 'Dr. Bob' DeMaria bring a wealth of knowledge from their professional work in the natural health field, as well as from their spiritual walk with God and marriage of 30 plus years into their teachings. It has been our privilege to know them for over 20 years and we believe them to be one of America's most inspiring couples, both in their informative books and videos and in their passionate and humorous speaking to large audiences across America. **We have heard their talk on sex and consider it 'the naked truth' no holds barred!** *They truly live out what they write and teach about and are an inspiration to everyone they meet. Their zest for life and for keeping the passion alive in their marriage is evident in everything they say and do. We are proud to call them friends and partners in ministry!"*

Marriage Authors, Paul & Patti Endrei
Glue, Sticking Power for Lifelong Marriages

"We were honored to have Dr. Bob and Debbie speak to our church congregation. The people enjoyed their humorous, inspiring and transforming messages. The life changing revelation on how a great sex life can transform marriages impacted our lives and brought our relationship to another level of deeper intimacy and fulfillment. Dr. Bob and Debbie are God's gift to this generation and beyond. We pray that millions of people around the world will discover these awesome kingdom principles as well." **Dr. David and Grace Kandole**
Global Outreach Christian Center

"The DeMarias are an exceptional couple. They are role models in their spiritual life, business prowess and especially in their marriage. Their oneness in relationship is unique among a generation of fragmented families. A must read to enhance and fulfill one's aspiration for a completed life!" **Pastor's Louis and Tina Kayatin**
Senior Pastors at Church on The North Coast

"Dr. Bob and Deb are the definition of over-comers in marriage, parenting, relationships and business. Their practical approach to life offers insight and real solutions to the dilemmas of our culture. In

D1372990

ministering to our multi-racial congregation, through honesty and humor, they always propel us to a new level of living."

Dr. Steve and Reita Ball Founders & Senior Pastors
Metro Tabernacle, Chattanooga, Tennessee

"My wife, Amira, and I have had the total privilege and honor to know and be friends with Dr. Robert and Debbie DeMaria.

"Throughout the past nine-plus years, we have seen a visible and living demonstration of a couple who continue to increase joy, love, and power in their marriage.

"Bob and Debbie's relationship is a light to all. It makes you want what they have!

"The health of their relationship is seen and felt by those who partake in getting to know them…They are truly a model of an ever increasing love affair. They are the best of friends, and they model marriage the way God intended it to be."

Pastor Dominic and Amira Russo
Oakland Christian Church, MI

Dr. Bob and Debbie's Guide to Sex and Romance:

Drugless Principles to Enhance Your Sex Life

Dr. Robert & Debbie DeMaria

Dr. Bob and Debbie's Guide to Sex and Romance:
Drugless Principles to Enhance Your Sex Life
by Robert & Debbie DeMaria

Published by:
Drugless Healthcare Solutions
P.O. Box 136
Avon, OH 44011

Phone:	(440) 323-3841
Fax:	(440) 322-2502
E-Mail:	druglesscare@aol.com
Web site:	www.DruglessDoctor.com

ISBN: 978-0-9728907-4-8

Printed in the United States of America
10 9 8 7 6 5 4 3 2 1

DISCLAIMER
This information is provided with the understanding that the author is not liable for the misconception or misuse of information included. Every effort has been made to make this material as complete and accurate as possible. The author of this material shall have neither liability nor responsibility to any person or entity with respect to any loss, damage or injury caused or alleged to be caused directly or indirectly by the information contained in this manuscript. The information presented herein is not intended to be a substitute for medical counseling.

Book cover design by Peri Poloni-Gabriel, Knockout Design, www.knockoutbooks.com
Page design by One-On-One Book Production, West Hills, CA

About Dr. Bob & Debbie DeMaria

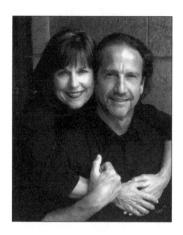

Dr. Bob and Debbie DeMaria have been married for over thirty years and have two wonderful sons that are the fruit of their marriage. Debbie has two Bachelor degrees, one is in Business Administration and the other is a Bachelor of Arts. She is a licensed minister and enjoys speaking and teaching with passion. Debbie and Dr. Bob coach and help people all around the world. Dr. Bob has a Bachelors degree in Human Biology. He has practiced clinically as a Chiropractor and consults with his second doctor degree; Doctor of Natural Health. He assists clients from around the world. Dr. Bob is the author of many books and the creator of the "Dr. Bob" series of wellness without medication. Dr. Bob and Deb host their own television program, and are guests on many local, national and global TV and radio programs.

ACKNOWLEDGMENTS

It is difficult to make something short and sweet and yet touch all the lives that have made this project possible or have been the encouragement behind the scenes.

First, to our sons, Dominic and Anthony. This has not always been an easy project for you to listen to but know you are the outcome of parents who loved not only you but each other.

To Dr. John and Karen Madiera, who listened to us from the very conception of this project to its final run! We pray we have made a difference in your lives too!

To Penny Novak, who was working with us in the earliest stages to bring life to our words — she knows our love oh too well!

To Janice Stringer, who also started with us way back until roadblocks and God's timing just didn't match.

Big thanks to Sarah DelliGatti. Sarah, without you we may still be on first base. You helped bring life to the mundane, and structure to the unstructured. Your were especially a big help with the Kid's and Women's Chapter, we appreciate your input.

We would be amiss to forget to thank the individuals who filled out the sex survey either online, at one of our talks, or at our office. We appreciate your openness, and frankness. You shared sorrows, struggles and victories, and we pray we addressed almost everything.

Thank you Holy Spirit for your perfect timing on this project. We know had it been when we desired, it may not have had the right material in it to touch our reader's lives.

TABLE OF CONTENTS

Appendices

We would like to introduce to you our dear friends:

We have known **Dr. Bob and Deb DeMaria** intimately for more than twenty years. As two of our closest friends, we have walked through some difficult times in life together and also have celebrated many victorious times. We have witnessed their marriage at very close range and seen them enjoy a devotion, closeness and intimacy with one another that few couples ever enjoy.

What they are about to share with you is not fantasy but real life. Their wisdom and knowledge on the subject of sex and sexual fulfillment is born out of their own romantic and sensual relationship, their extensive understanding of how the human body functions and how to fix both.

Dr. Bob and Deb are the real deal and know what they are talking about. It is our belief that your sex life will prosper as you glean and apply what you learn from these two amazing individuals.

Sincerely,

Dr. John and Karen Madeira

Author of *Setting Things Straight*

Introduction

Not every Christian leader's event gets as personal as one we attended some time ago. To make a point, one of the speakers asked the crowd what qualities most women look for in the ideal man. We weren't surprised to hear the women's answers: loving, kind, romantic, good-looking, and generous. Then the speaker asked the men in attendance what qualities they desired in the ideal woman. The overwhelming majority of men yelled out, "Sex!" The speaker asked for another quality and the men yelled even louder this time, "SEX!" Asked a third time, someone in the back responded, "Sex *all the time!*" I looked at my wife, Debbie, and whispered, "We need to get this book done *soon*."

As a couple with an incredibly satisfying sex life, we recognize a great need for marriages to have excitement and passion. We feel called to share the insight we've gained over thirty-two years of marriage that will restore, enhance, and heat up what's happening in your bedroom.

We meet tons of couples through our wellness practice, traveling and speaking engagements. It's usually pretty easy to tell which couples are enjoying a marriage filled with satisfying sexual intimacy. They smile at each other, touch often and communicate lovingly. On the other hand, we often see couples who criticize or contradict each other, rarely share eye contact, and whose body language screams, "Just leave me alone!" If they seem so distant in public, it's hard to imagine that they're any closer in the bedroom, or any room for that matter.

We've asked hundreds of couples to fill out marriage surveys for our use in writing this book and treating sexual dysfunction in our wellness practice. One godly Christian husband wrote down a comment that we've never forgotten. He penciled in the comment section, "My wife is always hot and ready!" This guy is 67; he and his wife have six kids, and they are obviously doing something right to make their marriage so sexually satisfying!

We desire the same for you and your spouse, and we want *both* of you to reap the rewards of being "hot and ready!" One of the great things about sex is that it can always be improved and even the learning and discovery can be enjoyable. (Think of time in your bedroom as the lab portion of this class!) The *journey* toward great sexual encounters can be as exciting and physically pleasurable as achieving the goal of incredible sex.

We've written this book for married couples who not only want their marriage to be Christ-centered, but who also want to have a wonderful, satisfying sex life and are willing to do whatever it takes to achieve that goal.

In talking with people who have walked through the pain and loss of divorce, we've never once heard someone say, "I left because the sex with my husband/wife was too good." Of course, good sex alone doesn't guarantee a blissful marriage, but the temperature in the bedroom is a pretty good indicator of the heat throughout the rest of a marriage. We've heard it said, "The grass is not greener on the other side, but it's just as hard to mow!" Why wander into other pastures when you can stay at home to water, weed and fertilize the spouse God has given you and enjoy the fruit that effort produces? You *can* wake up each morning looking forward to another day with the mate of your youth. We've been doing it ourselves for over thirty years.

As we mentioned before, Deb and I have been married since 1976. We were both in our early twenties and shortly after marrying moved away from our families so I could finish school. The distance from our families forced us to work out the conflicts of those first two years on our own. In 1976, during the country's bicentennial celebration, I purchased several rolls of quarters that had been manufactured as a commemoration of this special occasion. I figured at the time it would be a really neat gift to give Deb for our 25th anniversary. Talk about planning ahead! But that's how we've lived, without using the word divorce despite the conflicts and turmoil our marriage has faced. We've seen our share: alcohol addiction, money issues, child rearing, self employment, church turmoil, the aging and death of a parent and our own personal aging. Thankfully, God has faithfully encouraged, convicted and strengthened us year after year. I did give Deb those 1976 quarters on our 25th anniversary, along with an engraved plate. What a wonderful celebration of all that we had been through! Years later, we're even more passionately in love than we were then.

Deb and I have been involved in natural drugless healthcare since 1978, and we're excited to share with you how we've helped thousands in our practice experience restored health. Physical wellness is a <u>prerequisite</u> for sexual fulfillment, and God intends that we continue enjoying sex throughout our lifetimes. (Just imagine, Abraham was in his nineties and still going strong!) Our goal is to help you understand how the physiology of sex translates into actual lovemaking in your marriage.

Please understand that "lovemaking" doesn't necessarily mean "sex." Lovemaking is just what it sounds like: creating a feeling of love within your spouse. For men, lovemaking usually means the physical act of sexual intercourse. For most women, lovemaking has much more to do with romantic intimacy which may or may not include intercourse. We'll discuss both of these forms of lovemaking throughout the book.

We've met couples who are being challenged with different kinds of sexual impairments in various areas; I can tell you with absolute certainty these issues are not part of God's plan for your marriage. In fact, he wants your heart to throb *just thinking* about your spouse.[1]

You may be surprised by our candid confessions in this book. Some people are shocked when they hear us discussing sexuality, but they also admit to being very curious and intrigued by the subject matter. For example, the audience at one of our recent speaking engagements seemed reserved and quiet as we spoke but then returned the marriage questionnaire filled with incredibly intimate questions! Experiences like this have confirmed our suspicions *that people are desperate for sexual guidance* whether they're willing to admit it or not!

If your husband or wife coerced you into reading this book and you're feeling less than enthused about it, let us encourage you. Many partners who feel sexually frustrated simply walk out on a marriage. You've been blessed with a husband/wife who is walking in line with the Word of the Lord and has the courage to face some sexual issues head-on. That's great news! If you're still uncertain, browse the Table of Contents and start with a chapter that intrigues you. Your spouse will be moved by your willingness, and who knows — you might learn a thing or two!

At the end of each chapter we've included ideas for discussion. You may consider these points individually or as a couple, though we highly recommend coming together at some point to compare your responses. Finally, the end of the book has a section for notes. This is your chance to write your *own* chapter as you continue your sexual journey as a couple. Record your responses, struggles, sexual goals and anything else that's revealed during your reading time and intimate time together.

---

1   "In the night I dreamed that I sought the one whom I love…." Songs of Solomon 3:1

God created sex as a part of His wonderful plan for marriage and then called it "good." The One who planned it from the beginning can also be trusted to know exactly how it works best. Sex is biblical and a blessing. Man has twisted it and religion has made it naughty, but God's purposes still stand. Congratulations for having the courage to embark on a new romantic and sexual adventure with your spouse. We pray that God will bless you richly as you move into greater depths of love with Him and each other.

1
Burned Toast

Bob and I were traveling recently and had just settled into a beautiful bungalow when I stepped out into the hall and immediately noticed the smell of something burning. I couldn't quite put my finger on what the smell was but I knew it was familiar.

Later in the day we happened to run across an older Italian woman who was staying in the unit next to ours. While we were talking, I mentioned the odor I had smelled, and she went on to tell me in great detail where it had come from.

This city is famous for a specific kind of whole grain bread that is filled with all kinds of seeds and sprouts. To guarantee its freshness, it's only sold in half loaves. The woman loved this bread and had bought some that morning, putting fresh slices in the toaster. She stepped away to do other things until the smell of burning bread reminded her to return to the toaster. To her great disappointment, both pieces were charred. You and I probably would have thrown those pieces away, but this woman was unwilling to deny her taste buds and determined to save what she could. Knowing the richness of the bread was still there underneath the scarred, burned surface, she gently scraped the bread with a butter knife, her heart rejoicing to see the seeds and sprouts underneath still intact. She then buttered the toast and gently layered it with jelly. Looking at me with intensity in her voice and eyes, she exclaimed, "…and it was wonderful!" With the delight of a little girl she went on to tell me that now she had more bread to enjoy the next morning. This wonderful woman revealed a depth of wisdom and maturity as she spoke to me. Experience — and probably some tough times — had taught her to make the most of what she had and preserve everything available despite an outward appearance of uselessness.

As I listened to her story my mind wandered to our research for this book, and I couldn't stop thinking about what a wonderful object lesson the burned toast was. I sensed that my chance meeting with her was actually a divine appointment that would help communicate truth to our readers.

We've watched a number of couples become so distracted by life's demands that they neglect their marriages. It's not that they don't care or they intentionally damage the relationship, they just get disengaged with the allure of other things and think they'll get back to the relational stuff later when things slow down. As I'm sure you've already discovered, life never really quiets down! Before they know it, their marriage is in deep trouble.

The good news is most marriages — even deeply wounded ones — usually have some life left in them if the burned parts are gently scraped away. The bad news is our society believes that marriages are disposable, and divorce rates among Christian couples aren't much better than their non-Christian counter-parts. Even if a Christian couple knows the fundamentals of love and reconciliation, they are often tempted away from a troubled marriage by the desire of a "quick fix." They quickly jump at a divorce (throw away the burned toast) and set out in search of a newer, fresher relationship.

Bob and I believe that one reason our society is so quick to throw away marriages in the face of difficulty is a lack of strong family and ethnic ties. Bob's ancestry is Italian and mine is Polish and we both had the privilege of growing up in families with deep generational and marital bonds. Walking away from a marriage in our family would have also meant walking away from the amazing and supportive structure of extended family. The strength and stability of a marriage is not just a benefit for a husband and wife and their children; the blessings of that relationship flow out to grandparents, siblings, nieces, nephews and every other member of the extended family. Sadly, today's families are often scattered across the country, held together by birthday cards and occasional visits, continuously shattered, formed and reformed by divorce, remarriage and mixed families. Often there is no family depth and history of sound biblical advice, let alone a godly upbringing. It's understandable, then, that many couples are willing to throw away a burned and wounded relationship instead of investing the time necessary to bring healing and wholeness. Many times they simply aren't aware there's a better way.

The marriage assessments we conducted revealed that many couples have thought seriously about discarding their marriages. You may be in a marriage of ten, twenty or even thirty years and at times feel like it would be easier to throw it away and start again with someone new. Scraping off the charred parts of your marriage (wounds, conflict, etc.) probably doesn't sound very enticing, and to be honest, it's hard work! Sometimes throwing away the whole thing seems like the easiest way out of a bad situation. But the truth is that you and your spouse are spiritually one flesh, and pulling flesh apart is never an easy process; it's painful, bloody and heart-wrenching. In the long run, the wounds caused by divorce are even more horrible than the unpleasant task of scraping away the old hurts and searching for a bit of life in what's left of a marriage.

After scraping the bread, this sweet little old lady buttered what was left of each piece. Once you've determined to work on your marriage and remove its most ugly pieces, it's time to butter your relationship with the healing oil of the Holy Spirit! Every marriage relationship needs a continuous fresh anointing from God, which gives us grace for each other and smoothes over the rough places. Isaiah 10:27 says, "It shall come to pass in that day that his burden will be taken away from your shoulder, and his yoke will be destroyed because of the anointing oil."[1]

The anointing of God brings healing and restoration. It fills us with the compassion and grace we need to forgive each other on a daily basis. God's word is very clear about the importance of the oil of forgiveness. Mark 11:26 states, "But if you do not forgive, neither will your Father in heaven forgive your failings and short-comings." This command doesn't exclude forgiving your spouse!

Many people have a misguided view of forgiveness; they believe that forgiving is giving in to their spouse and "losing" the fight. Nothing could be further from the truth! Forgiveness grows out of the humble understanding that I, too, have faults and will at some point turn to you with a sorrowful face to say, "I'm sorry. Will *you* forgive *me*?" Allow the oil of God's anointing to bring healing into your marriage through the redemptive act of forgiveness.

After spreading butter on the toast, the woman added jelly. What a wonderful flavor it must have added to that bread! We have the opportunity to add flavoring to our marriages by the words we speak. Colossians 4:6 says, "Let your speech at all times be gracious (pleasant and winsome), seasoned (as it were) with salt, (so that you may never be at a loss)."

The words we speak are so important; they have the power to bring life or death to our relationships.[2] Speaking positive, encouraging words is like adding salt to a delicious feast — it brings out the flavor of each food. Too often couples choose to

---

1   From the New King James Version.
2   Proverbs 18:21

encourage and edify those outside their home while speaking only negative and critical words to their own families! Because we realize how destructive this habit can be, Bob and I have made a quiet agreement you may want to incorporate into your own life. We've committed to never demean one another, whether in our own private conversations or especially while speaking with others. This is not an easy task when we're sharing with close, intimate friends, yet we realize that once words are spoken they can never be taken back. Those words become planted in the minds of both speaker and listener and are forever available to be rewound and replayed.

I'm very thankful that the Lord laid this principle on my heart when I was very young. Bob and I started dating in high school and six years later we were married. Those six years were sometimes rocky and filled with the anguish of teenage love. During that time, my intuition told me not to share our struggles with my parents. I knew they wouldn't hesitate to take my side, and I felt strongly that Bob and I would eventually be together. When that happened, I wanted them to think highly of him and not let what I'd shared get in the way of their love for and acceptance of him as a son-in-law. I'm thrilled to tell you that my parents adore Bob and are some of his greatest supporters, but it could have been much different if I'd shared without restraint.

That wonderful lady's toast turned out to be everything she had hoped for. Despite being burned it still had value, tasted delicious, and was the solution to her hunger and longing. It was worth the effort as she savored each bite. Your marriage is no different! Determine to salvage what is good, scrape away what's wounded, bring healing with God's anointing oil, and flavor your relationship with words seasoned with grace. Your relationship *can* be all you dream of if you'll give God the chance to work in you and through you for His glory.

JUST TELL ME WHAT TO DO:

☐ Consider recording your responses to each chapter in a journal.

☐ Evaluate your marriage separately using not only the principles but the bullet points from this chapter. Then come together as a couple to discuss these. Are there ways you've been neglecting your marriage? Are there distractions in your life that should be set aside so you can once again make your marriage your highest priority?

☐ Reminisce about your past positive experiences as a couple. What made those times so good? Do you give your marriage the same tender attention today that you were on the days those memories were created?

☐ Are there significant parts of your relationship that have been tossed aside because they seem burned and useless? How can you start the process of scraping away those negative habits? Consider a professional Christian counselor if the task seems overwhelming.

☐ What challenges have you already overcome? Rejoice in those victories!

☐ Release yourselves to the work of the Holy Spirit. Communicate to Him your willingness to listen to His voice and obey what He calls each of you to do for the healing and restoration of your marriage.

☐ Ask the Holy Spirit to pour forgiveness into your hearts.

☐ Commit to speaking only words that affirm and encourage your spouse.

2
The Hunt

"he Hunt" is a phrase I've coined to describe the pursuit of your goals. In particular, the goals regarding your marriage. I have a mental picture of hunters using their skills in the great outdoors to track and capture their prey. It's a task they relish and enjoy, a sport that makes use of all their skill and weaponry. Trophy or no trophy, they live for the thrill of the hunt.

Your pursuit of your spouse should be equally thrilling. Notice that I didn't say, "Your pursuit of sex...." No, the highest goal in marriage is the pursuit of *intimacy*, and that looks different for each person in every marriage. A spouse whose sole focus is the meeting of his own needs is missing out on the greatest prize of marriage: the mind, heart, soul and body of their partner. It's a wonderful irony that pursuing the fulfillment of your spouse's needs generally guarantees the fulfillment of your own. The Hunt is on!

It would be nice if men and women had the same needs when it comes to intimacy. I believe God intentionally designed us with differing needs and strengths so that we'd have a deep craving for our partner. In his book *The Purpose and Power of Love and Marriage*, my good friend Myles Monroe puts forth the five significant needs of men and women. We'll address each in turn.

Men	Women
Continuous need for sexual fulfillment	Cyclical need for sexual fulfillment
Recreational companionship	Affection and communication
Attractiveness leading to feelings of love	Honesty leading to feelings of trust
Domestic support of wife	Financial support of husband
Wife's respect	Husband's commitment

SEXUAL FULFILLMENT

The greatest physical need of a healthy man is sexual fulfillment. If you don't believe me, just ask your husband what he is thinking about a good percentage of the time! His body is wired to crave sex about every 48 to 72 hours.[1] Ladies, you can either bemoan this continual need or be thankful that his desire is directed toward *you*. It's one significant way God draws couples together who might otherwise drift apart due to the demands of our busy lives. Women's sexual drives are cyclical, based on their hormone and fertility levels.

RECREATIONAL COMPANIONSHIP

Men want a partner, not just in bed, but in almost every aspect of their lives. Ladies, if your husband enjoys a particular sport you can bless him immensely by learning more about it and joining him. This will give you lots of time and opportunity for….

AFFECTION AND COMMUNICATION

Gentlemen, your wife craves the easy affection and conversation of a lover and a friend. This includes holding hands, hugging, kissing and snuggling. Such affectionate gestures don't always imply that she wants to have sex but can certainly become part of foreplay as her feelings of love grow through your gentle

---

1   This is generally the amount of time it takes for a man's body to replenich its supply of sperm and seminal fluid.

touches. Women also long to talk with their husbands about more than the children and the budget. Ask how her day went and what tomorrow holds. Pray with her and for her. Encourage her dreams and goals. Don't come home, sit on the sofa with the paper and grunt your way through dinner. Engage her!

ATTRACTIVENESS

Men want to feel sexually attracted to their spouses. This *doesn't* mean a woman has to look like a runway model, but women should pursue their husbands by offering their very best. Maintain personal hygiene, invest in up-to-date clothing, have your hair styled and consider what will appeal to your spouse. If he likes makeup, wear it. Ask him to help you choose a nice perfume.[2]

On the other hand, men need to be understanding regarding this subject. A mother who has just delivered a new baby and isn't getting any rest is lucky if her socks match! As long as you have grace for each other and are determined to act selflessly instead of selfishly, this need can be balanced to benefit both of you.

HONESTY

Women need to know they can rely on their husband's word. This includes being home when you say you will be home, being open about your feelings on intimate matters and straight-forward during disagreements. All of these communicate that you care about her and that she can trust you.

DOMESTIC SUPPORT

Please don't turn away from this important discussion because of its title. I know "domestic" has gained a bad reputation in recent years, but I truly believe that this is an important need for most

---

2   Proverbs 27:9 says, "Perfume and incense bring joy to the heart…

men. Simply stated, men want to come home to a haven, and women are generally the caretakers of the home whether they work as well or not. A man wants to feel like the king of his castle, and wise men will treat their wives like a queen to bring this about! Some men really treasure a hot dinner each night, while others value a neat and tidy house. Ladies, find out what moves your husband and do your best to provide it. Solicit help from the children and make him feel like a king when he walks in the door. You're likely to get more help clearing the dinner table if you graciously meet this vital need!

FINANCIAL SUPPORT

This is another hot button topic in our society as many women bring home just as much money as their male counterparts do. Still, it brings great security to most women to know that their husbands take the role of provider seriously. If she were unable to work, would you graciously take over the complete financial support of the family? This becomes a reality for more and more families as women choose to stay home with newborns and preschoolers. Men commonly find great satisfaction in work, and God was wise in giving them the job of provider while blessing women to be strong nurturers. As you each embrace your particular roles, needs will be met and your whole family will be blessed.

RESPECT

Individuals greatly desire the respect and admiration of their spouse. This is a biblical directive that too often bows to our culture's notion that respect must be earned. Both husbands and wives are to respect their married partner regardless of their behavior. Ladies, would you want your husband to only love you when are acting lovable?! It's entirely possible to respect him while disagreeing with some of his actions. Look for the goodness in him; seek out ways to express gratitude and respect. Thank him for being a diligent worker and a good dad. Encourage him instead of nagging. Praise him in front of the children and your friends.

Husbands, you would be wise to honor your wife with compliments and kind gestures. Be the kind of man she can easily respect. This means being a gentleman and treating her like a lady. It means putting away immature schoolboy behavior like inappropriate language and unnecessary jokes.

COMMITMENT

Jokes have been made about men's fear of commitment, but this is an important need for women. Women need to know that you are in your marriage for the long haul. They need reassurance of your love long after their beauty has faded and their "self talk" significance may have dwindled. When the world would cast them aside, they long to hear that you will be by their side, still holding their hand and continuing on the journey you've started. In quiet moments, tell your wife how much you enjoy being with her. Make it fun. Never give her any reason to doubt your level of commitment.

Zig Ziglar, one of the greatest speakers in our generation, says, "You can get anything in life that you want if you help enough people get exactly what they want." It's the absolute truth! If you're only focused on meeting your own needs, good luck to you. It's only as you pursue your *spouse's* needs that intimacy will grow in your marriage. Increased intimacy means better sex — and lots more of it! The blessing that outweighs it all is a wonderful marriage to your very best friend that will endure everything life can throw at you.

Deb and I regularly receive compliments on how well we treat each other. We are genuinely best friends and it has become natural to act with love and thankfulness towards each other. We extend the same courtesy to each and every person we come into contact with, whether clerks at a gas station, the dry cleaner, waiter or waitress, or the barista at our favorite coffee house. This understanding of the value of people (including each other) creates a magnetism that's contagious. It fills us with admiration for each other, makes our day easier, and increases our desire for sex. Putting smiles on the faces of everyone around you is one of the easiest ways to impact your marriage and the world!

A man in Luke 11:9 was tenacious as he pleaded with his neighbor for bread to feed visiting house guests. I engage in The Hunt the very same way: I'm relentless in my daily pursuit of Deb. I'm not only nice when I want to have sex with her. (Those of you who try to turn on the charm for those moments know how far it gets you: Nowhere!) Women can see through your manipulation and it's incredibly harmful to a marriage to behave in this manner. No, you should always be tenderly knocking on the door of your lover's heart, looking for ways to meet their needs and bless them. Trust me, serving your spouse selflessly will ultimately open the door to their body as well as the doors to their heart, mind and soul!

Sometimes The Hunt turns into a sexual rendezvous and sometimes it doesn't. Either way is fine because I know I'm pursuing my wife as God intends and priming the pump for when she is ready to be intimate. And ladies, I don't want to leave you out of The Hunt. You should be just as focused on meeting your husband's needs as he is meeting yours. This will mean serving him sexually when you aren't exactly jumping for joy. Every sexual encounter doesn't have to be full of earthquakes and fireworks; On-In-and-Out-Sex (which some may call a "quickie") is a wonderful tool for serving your husband when you're tired or busy or just plain not interested. I will tell you, though, that your husband will just go crazy at those times when you approach him wanting nothing more than a wild romp or a long, intimate encounter.

My Hunt for Deb normally starts every morning when the alarm goes off. I tell Deb that I love her each morning as well as multiple other times during the day. I fix her coffee just the way she likes it: piping hot with organic cream, in a cup with a closed lid. Find out what your spouse likes, down to the details, and do your best to provide it. It's very special to me that few people in the world know Deb as I do, and she feels valued that I care about the little things. Don't assume that you know — ask!

We pray together each morning and take turns reading a devotional, then spend some individual quiet time in our Bibles. We jog and ride our bikes together and then get ready for the day. The whole process takes about three hours starting at 4:30 in the morning, three days a week. On most other days, we "sleep in" until six. This schedule works for us and allows us wonderful time to pursue each other. Your Hunt will look as unique as you are. The important thing is that you find ways to pursue each other, planning time to meet each other's needs and develop deepening intimacy in your marriage. Schedule time for shared activities, communication, spiritual growth, and sexual intimacy. I've observed couples who are over-involved in church activities and neglect their marriage as a result. Don't grow so busy with the outside world that you forget The Hunt for the heart of your spouse.

TEAMWORK

A huge part of The Hunt that I would like to bring to light is the role of a helper/partner. As a couple, you were brought together to fulfill certain purposes in each of your lives. Spouses should be helping each other to fulfill their God-ordained destiny instead of living separate lives. It may not seem that romantic to help your wife fold laundry, but if she was called to be a homemaker, you are encouraging her to walk in that calling. (You are also increasing your chances of "getting lucky," but as I stated before, that's a secondary goal to capturing your wife's heart!) Ladies, has your husband chosen a challenging career? Helping him get it together in the morning with projects, computers, day planners and lunch may not sound so glamorous, but you are a co-laborer helping him walk out his calling. The role of a helper is so vital to a happy marriage and is often overlooked by the world. It's one of the easiest ways to serve your spouse and put a smile on their face each and every day. *Ask* what you can do to be a blessing to your partner in small and simple ways.

I make my own breakfast and prepare healthy snacks to take to the office while Deb is upstairs getting ready in the morning. I don't want her to feel like she is my "personal attendant." When our sons were young I also made their breakfast as often as possible during the week and then on the weekends. I wanted to teach them to be responsible and not expect a woman to cater to their every need. They picked up on my example and some lucky ladies will thank me for it after they've married our sons!

I often carry the laundry basket to our room for Deb and take it back to the laundry room when it's filled. I wipe up the bathroom sink after I shower and shave and return my towels to their rack rather than dropping them on the floor. Dirty clothes go in the hamper and I iron my own pants, creased at the hanger line. I rinse my dishes in the sink before putting them in the dishwasher. I'm not telling you this to boast; the list of what Deb does for me is equally long and impressive. She maintains our home, our personal calendar and appointments, travel plans, food, and is administrator of my offices as well as Chief Financial Officer. She helps me set up for talks and events and keeps my life in order as well as taking care of all kinds of personal details for both of us and sometimes even for our sons. She schedules couple time for us and then considers how to meet my most intimate needs by making herself visually attractive according to what she knows I like. The point is, we *serve each other* and *don't keep score* of who's doing more. We simply look for ways to be on The Hunt for each other's hearts.

We take turns making lunch depending on our schedules. Deb normally makes dinner, but on the days I'm available, I grill outside. In the spring, I bring fresh lilacs home for Deb because they remind her of her grandparents and I know she loves them. Here's a gem: on a country drive one day we came across the most beautiful deep purple lilacs. She was just raving over these flowers, so I stopped the car, walked up to the house and asked if they wouldn't mind if I cut my wife some of their lilacs. After they recovered from the initial shock of seeing such a giddy, loving couple ooohing and aaahing over the flowers, they said to help myself. Deb was grinning from ear to ear, and you can bet I had a huge smile on my face that night as a result! No, I didn't do it to get her into bed, but that was a wonderful byproduct of pursuing her heart. I did it because I'm constantly on The Hunt for Deb's heart, mind *and* her body. It's impossible to get just one without the others, contrary to what many men believe. If you only capture your wife's body, you haven't captured her at all and she'll only resent you for treating her as an object. Be on The Hunt for *all* of her and you'll get everything you've ever dreamed of in a friend and lover.

In the Message translation of the Bible, 1 Corinthians 6:16 – 7:1 says it this way: "There's more to sex than mere skin on skin. Sex is as much spiritual mystery as physical fact. As written in Scripture, 'The two become one.' Since we want to become spiritually one with the Master, we must not pursue the kind of sex that avoids commitment and intimacy, leaving us more lonely than ever—the kind of sex that can never 'become one'."

I'm afraid many men don't really understand this concept. They believe that sex is a right instead of a privilege. If you're smart, start spending as much time considering how to meet your wife's needs as you presently spend trying to get your own met. The dividends are priceless!

Hunting your spouse means you'll have to be on the lookout for all of the little clues they leave. This reminds me of how a hunter tracks his prey, watching for every sign of their presence. Does he mention that he likes his shirts pressed a certain way? Aha! A clue as to how best to Hunt him! Does she sigh every time she puts the children to bed without your help? A useful piece of information for any man who wants to capture his wife's heart! If you're unsure what to do, ASK!!! Any spouse would be delighted to hear, "Honey, how can I show you I love you today?"

Want some ideas to start with? Here are a few:

MEN:

➤ Empty the garbage can when you see it's getting full.

➤ Rinse your dinner dishes and run the garbage disposal.

➤ Say "I love you!" often and sincerely.

➤ Empty the dishwasher or dry the dishes for your wife.

➤ Get a new box of tissues when you use the last one.

➤ Do the same for the toilet paper and find out if she likes the roll dispensed over or under.

➤ Help her put the kids to bed. Better yet, do it yourself and give her a break.

➤ Kiss her for no reason at all.

➤ Put down the lid!

➤ Fill up the gas tank in the car.

➤ Rinse your toothpaste out of the sink.

➤ Clean out the tub or shower when you're done.

➤ Leave a short love note where you know she'll find it during the day.

➤ Help make the bed in the morning.

➤ Help her carry the groceries in from the car.

LADIES:

- Make a hot breakfast for him on the weekend.
- Buy a new piece of lingerie and wear it for him.
- Try out a new shade of lipstick.
- Let him see you making an effort to exercise.
- Praise him in front of the children or your friends.
- Buy a new outfit for a night out.
- Approach him for sex and ask if there's something he's especially desired.
- Send him a sexy text message on his personal cell phone.
- Pick up the house a bit before he gets home.
- Thank him for being a hard worker and provider.
- Learn the rules of his favorite sport and watch the next game with him.
- Get a new hairstyle just to surprise him.
- Put on perfume even when you're not going out.

Husbands, when you don't help your wife during the day, having sex becomes just one more thing on her To Do List. Instead, help her finish the list and be able to enjoy making love with a clear, unhurried mind. Ladies, making love to your husband (even a quickie) will make him more open to regular affection and communication. Do you see how the "Hunt" for your spouse's heart leads to the "Meeting" of your own needs?

The right perspective makes all the difference in how you approach your spouse and the quality of your marriage. Start Hunting for each other in small and large ways today! Determine to be the person who captures your spouse's heart, mind and body.

JUST TELL ME WHAT TO DO

❑ Discuss the five significant needs of men and women from the table at the beginning of the chapter. Do you recognize any of them in your own life?

❑ Be honest with yourself and each other: Have you been seeking to meet your spouse's needs or your own? What needs to change so that you're on The Hunt for your partner instead of yourself?

❑ Wives, have you taken seriously your husband's need for sexual fulfillment?

❑ Husbands, have you been patient with your wife's cyclical need for sexual intimacy?

❑ Is there an activity you can enjoy together?

❑ Are there ways you can be more affectionate (without the goal of sex in mind)?

❑ Do you spend time talking about goals and dreams? Do you actively listen to your spouse?

❑ Are you maintaining a healthy, attractive body that brings pleasure to your spouse?

❑ Are you honest and truthful with each other?

❑ Ladies, are you treating your husband like the king of his castle? Husbands, are you treating your wife like a queen? What can you do to make this a reality in your home?

❑ Husbands, do you take the role of provider seriously?

❑ Wives, are you showing respect to your husband by building him up, or are you belittling him and tearing him down? What changes can you make so that he sees and hears your respect for him?

❑ Gentleman, can your wife fully rest in your commitment to her? Do you send mixed messages by looking at other women or acting inappropriately? Assure her of your love and commitment daily.

❑ Are you helping each other fulfill God's call on your lives? Are you seeking small ways to bless your spouse? Browse the list again and choose one or two ways to start.

❑ Look at your calendars and determine if outside interests are robbing you of quality intimate time together. What activities should be limited to guarantee couple time for the two of you?

❑ Start praying together and find a church to attend if you aren't already. Involve the whole family in your spiritual journey.

3
Hormones

Hormones act as messengers in the body, and the endocrine (or glandular) system plays a critical role in sexual desire and the ability to respond physically to those needs. The endocrine system is made up of eight different glands located strategically throughout the body.

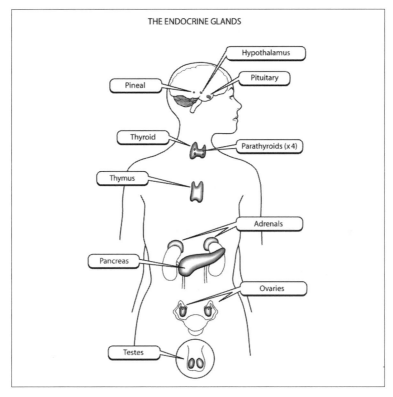

THE ENDOCRINE GLANDS

Gland	Location	Function
Hypothalamus	Brain	CEO of hormone system
Ovaries	A pair found in the lower abdomen	Produce progesterone and estrogen. Release eggs or ovum.
Testes	A pair found outside of the body	Produce testosterone and sperm
Adrenal	A pair located on top of the kidneys	Produce multiple hormones, including sex hormones
Pancreas	Located in the mid abdomen	Creates insulin and enzymes
Thyroid	Mid throat area	Produces thyroid hormone
Parathyroid	Adjacent to thyroid tissue	Assists in calcium function
Pineal	Brain	Controls waking and sleeping patterns
Pituitary	Base of the brain	Secretes many leading hormone activators

In addition to these major glands, the endocrine system includes pockets of hormone-producing cells in the small intestines, heart, kidneys and stomach. The endocrine glands and other systems work together to maintain health and proper sexual function.

HYPOTHALAMUS

The hypothalamus is the CEO of the hormonal system and the Commander-in-Chief of sexual activity. While it may feel as though sexual needs originate in your body, sex actually starts in the mind. Most men are initially stimulated visually while women become aware of sexual feelings as a response to romantic thoughts and gestures. These sights and feelings arouse the emotions and the hypothalamus releases hormones to activate other glands in the body, connecting sexual thoughts with physical responses to ready the body for sexual intimacy.

OVARIES and TESTES

The ovaries are a pair of reproductive glands found in the abdomen of females. The ovaries release eggs and produce hormones, including estrogen and progesterone. Similarly, the testes are a pair of reproductive glands found in males. They are cradled in the scrotum and hang outside of the body, where they produce sperm and testosterone. The term "gonad" refers to the ovaries in females and testes in males.

ADRENAL

You have two adrenal glands, located on the top of each kidney. They serve many functions including affecting the size of the pupils, instrumental in the ability to ejaculate in men, and producing steroids including sex hormones, pain-relieving cortisol and mineral regulating ligament-strengthening hormones. I very commonly see patients whose adrenal glands are over-worked and exhausted.[1] A common body signal of this exhaustion is sensitivity to bright light. Wearing sunglasses because of adrenal stress prevents the full spectrum of light from reaching the back of the eye complicating your optimal health puzzle.

PANCREAS

The pancreas produces insulin and enzymes for proper digestion and metabolism and can be overworked when the diet is full of processed foods.

Packaged devitalized foods have been stripped of nutrients, resulting in increased stress on the pancreas to make up for insufficient enzyme levels.

---

1   Adrenal gland exhaustion is discussed in detail in the Adrenal Gland Chapter.

THYROID and PARATHYROID

The thyroid receives messages from the pituitary gland and creates thyroid hormones, which are used by all the cells of the body. The thyroid sets the pace for optimal metabolism. The parathyroid works in conjunction with the thyroid to aid in proper calcium metabolism.

PINEAL

This tiny gland is incredibly significant but rarely discussed by health care professionals. It is linked to the hypothalamus and is influenced by diet and nutrition. The pineal gland produces and secretes melatonin in response to light rays from the sun and those reflected off the moon, creating the cycle of waking and sleeping.

I've consulted many patients who struggle with a condition called Seasonal Affective Disorder, or S.A.D., which closely mimics depression. This disorder occurs late in summer as the seasons are changing and the hours of daylight are rapidly declining. These patients tend to be women who are also experiencing emotional struggles at this time of year as their "babies" are starting kindergarten, older children are returning to school, or they are sending teens off to college. The combination of emotional challenges and changing sleep and wake cycles can be overwhelming, and I've found S.A.D. to be a result of these struggles as well as stress and nutritional deficiencies. It's very common for these patients to experience a decreased sex drive as well. I recommend using a product called phosphatydylcholine and taking up to nine a day. Phosphatydylcholine is very useful in stabilizing emotional health when challenged in the fall by Seasonal Affective Disorder.

PITUITARY

The pituitary gland is nearly as significant as the hypothalamus. Once it receives orders from the CEO, it conveys the messages to several glands and tissues critical to sexual function including the ovaries and testes, adrenal glands and thyroid. The pituitary also plays a major role in metabolism, digestion and growth by influencing the autonomic nervous system.

After taking a closer look at these glands, I hope you realize how amazing and important your endocrine system is. Sexual thoughts would progress no further were it not for this system of hormone messengers preparing your body for action. Unfortunately, I see an epidemic of patients whose endocrine systems are overworked, stressed, and nutritionally starving. When a patient complains of a lack of sexual desire, it's almost always because their endocrine system is exhausted and near collapse. Other symptoms of hormonal burnout include chronic degenerative diseases like diabetes, high blood pressure and whole body inflammation with elevated cholesterol. These three conditions alone are responsible for most of the asexual marriages and resulting marital challenges I've treated.

Young couples generally start out with high libidos, often desiring to have sex daily and even multiple times each day. Sexual desire usually wanes for most women after children are born and during the intensive baby and toddler years. Unfortunately, many women report that it never really returns, to the dismay of both husband and wife. Other patients may have some desire but no ability to physically respond to their intentions. It's not at all uncommon for me to consult with women in their twenties who are experiencing tender breasts, a dry vagina and a heavy menstrual flow, all the while taking psychoactive medications. The last thing they feel like doing is having sex, and due to poor cellular health, they're not capable of having it anyway!

Women aren't the only ones suffering from hormonal imbalance; I see plenty of men in my practice who quietly admit to decreased or non-existent sexual desire and erectile dysfunction complications. It's been my experience that most of these patients are physically exhausted, drained from poor diets, over-indulging in alcohol, abusing recreational and prescription drugs, smoking cigarettes and experiencing daily pressure from their jobs. Many of them are taking one or more psychoactive prescription medications just to take the edge off.

Many couples report having intercourse only once or twice a month, and others are experiencing no sexual intimacy at all. Your body *can* get along without sex to survive; just ask anyone who looks exhausted. The sad news is, most marriages are hard pressed to *passionately* survive without sex, especially when one partner is feeling unable or unwilling to perform and the other is growing increasingly resentful of their withering intimate life.

Deb and I both strongly believe that this **doesn't have to be the norm** for married couples. We are both over fifty years old, have been married for over thirty years and are still having passionate sex *without* the use of pills and jellies. We believe this is possible for *every couple* who commits to a healthy lifestyle!

The endocrine system is probably the first part of your body to be impacted by nutritional deficiencies. Sexual functions are affected just as much by nutrition as they are by physical and emotional health. Thankfully, nutritional changes are relatively simple to make and the effects are almost immediate. Instead of masking sexual problems by taking prescription drugs (and causing a whole host of side effects that must be dealt with), you have the ability to radically improve your health and the sexual health of your marriage by making small changes in your diet and lifestyle.

Your body makes hormones from the food you eat. Healthy, organic whole foods result in healthy hormone production. Conversely, toxic foods full of sugar, taste enhancers, preservatives and trans fats will result in inadequate hormone production and a body that is literally starving for nutrition. Many of you reading this book are suffering from hormonal imbalance and lowered libidos and the reason is as close as your kitchen pantry. If you're consuming a diet full of nutritionally-deficient processed foods and are addicted to sweets, soft drinks, and calorie-laden meals, your body is doing its best with what you're feeding it, but it's not functioning anywhere close to its peak!

If you recognize some of the symptoms of hormonal exhaustion discussed in this chapter, I strongly suggest you read the Adrenal Chapter and commit to making healthy changes in your diet and lifestyle. Your body will thank you, your sex drive will increase, and you and your spouse will find renewed passion and excitement as you travel this journey toward health and healing together.

JUST TELL ME WHAT TO DO

- ❏ Your endocrine system requires whole foods to operate at top efficiency. Start eliminating processed food from your diet and get your nutrients from organic whole foods.

- ❏ High lignan, organic flax oil is a great way to start improving overall hormonal health. You should take one tablespoon per one hundred pounds of body weight.

- ❏ Plan your meals with the entire family and eat together as often as possible to create healthy eating habits in your children that will last a lifetime.

- ❏ Eliminate sugar from your diet to avoid stressing the adrenal glands.

4

Frolicking Fundamentals for Men

If you're a typical man, the amount of sex you're actually having doesn't satisfy your sexual appetite. While libidos vary between individuals, men typically have higher sexual appetites than women. (This is more understandable when you consider that a sexual experience almost *always* results in climax for men, while the odds for women walking away sexually satisfied are much lower.) An unfortunate consequence of sexual frustration for men is that they often feel like any intimacy that occurs is at the whim of their wife. But the truth is that husbands have an incredible amount of control over the frequency of sexual intimacy within their marriage *if they are willing to be considerate lovers who are concerned with their wife's needs as well as their own!*

Would you like to have more sexually intimate times with your wife? I'd like to suggest some things you can do that will guarantee her willingness — and eagerness! — to have sex with you. The first is what you offer her with your own body. It's amazing to me how many men don't stop to consider their appearance. They have high standards for their wives (makeup, clothing, etc.) but take very little time to consider what *they* are bringing to the bedroom. I have one patient who confided in me that her husband constantly picks *and eats* the scabs off his skin. Are you surprised that it makes her cringe to think of being intimate with him? I'm not! So let's take an honest look at something men far too often overlook: personal hygiene.

Do you get a haircut regularly? Trim nose and ear hair? Keep your nails clean and trimmed? I know a woman whose husband is a contractor. He's a hard worker and it shows on his hands. She told me it was actually painful when he ran his hands over her body because they were so torn up. Instead of reacting in frustration every time he scraped his hands across her skin, this woman prayed for wisdom in responding to her husband. God faithfully answered, directing her to tenderly care for her husband's hands. Now she occasionally washes his hands, exfoliates them with a natural scrub and rubs lotion into them. Not only does it solve the problem, but it's become an occasional part of their foreplay. Her husband enjoys the tender attention and this wonderful wife receives a spiritual blessing. She could chose to complain and turn down her husband's advances, leading to his resentment and frustration. Instead, she blesses her husband and in turn, their marriage. What a difference her godly response makes!

Do you shave regularly? Whiskers can actually burn a woman's sensitive skin, especially if you have gray facial hair which is extremely coarse. Facial hair means less area to shave, but you should consider what impact it might be having on your sex life. In fact, have you ever thought to ask your wife if she even likes your mustache and/or beard? If I knew my wife would be more attracted to me and want more sex if I had a handlebar mustache, you can bet I'd start growing one today! But if facial hair bothers her, shave regularly. The benefits are worth a few more minutes in front of the mirror.

A large part of personal hygiene is your body odor. Your body could radiate a pungent fragrance; it should be a *pleasant* one! Do you shower daily? Women have a very keen sense of smell; they are much more sensitive than men. I can't think of anything less appealing than having a sweaty, smelly naked spouse trying to wrap themselves around me. Before you approach your wife, make sure you have showered and put on deodorant and clean clothes.

Speaking of body aroma, women are also very concerned about their own personal hygiene, specifically their vaginal scent. Vaginas are not fragrance-free, hormonal changes and your wife's level of physical activity all contributes to the way it radiates its own fragrance. If your wife feels embarrassed by her scent, find ways to help her carve out time for a shower or a bath. Put the kids to bed while she freshens up. She will be thankful for your help and it will give her time to relax and get in the mood. If it's possible, join her in the shower and offer to scrub her back. (the shower is a great place for occasional On, In and Out sex if you don't have much time, and it allows her to quickly wash up afterward.)

Do your feet reek? Mine used to when I consumed alcohol and my liver and kidney function was compromised. How is your breath? Chronic bad breath can be a sign of poor digestion. Stop drinking fluids with your meals, as too much liquid will dilute the enzymes in your stomach and interfere with digestion. As that food sits putrefying in your stomach it releases gases that can lead to bad breath. Talk to your natural health care provider for advice on a natural digestive aid. And by the way, I would not use sugar or sugar substitute-based breath fresheners. They will compromise your adrenal gland function as discussed in the Adrenal Chapter.

Do you smoke or chew tobacco? If you do, you're asking your wife to kiss a chimney! You can imagine the damper that puts on her desire to be intimate with you.

While we're talking about smells, it may be time to update your cologne. Do you still have the same old bottle from five years ago? It's probably stale by now. Set up a date with your wife and go shopping together for a new scent. You'd spend money on a game of golf, fishing tackle, or any other hobby you may have; why not invest in your sex life? Cologne is an easy way to help put your lady in the mood or at least help her start thinking about it. You should purchase one ounce *spray* bottles because the oil on your skin as well as contaminants on your fingers can alter the scent of cologne that must be applied by hand. Go to a men's store, a large department store or a specialty store where the products are fresh and purchase a new fragrance.

Is your wardrobe clean, neat, and well put together? You don't have to turn into a GQ model, and that's probably not even what your wife wants. But I can guarantee she will appreciate a well-dressed man and be more open to sex if you approach her clean and looking great!

Even more important than wooing your wife physically is meeting her emotional desires. Men who are focused on their own needs while ignoring their spouse's desires are understandably going to get turned down again and again. But when you consider her and make her requests your priority, she will be more likely to respond sexually.

Are you listening to your wife? Putting down the paper, turning off the TV, turning away from the computer and really listening? If you aren't, don't expect her to listen to your pleas for intimacy; she is feeling ignored and unloved. In the morning, ask about her plans for the day. In the evening, remember those plans and ask how they went. Trust me, she will immediately recognize and appreciate that you remembered what she had going on during the day! Talk about more than business as usual subjects: the kids, the house, the calendar, her job. What are her dreams? What is God speaking to her about lately? Let her know you are interested in every aspect of her life.

Another important need you should be meeting for your wife is quality time together. She wants more than your paycheck and an occasional romp in the bedroom — she wants *you*! That means carving out time for just the two of you, write it down in your calendar, you should be doing it! You will undoubtedly be hoping that a date night will include sex, but don't pressure her in that regard. Just enjoy spending time together. If it leads to sex, great; if it doesn't, you've still made an investment in your marriage that will pay off in the future.

One of the easiest ways to bless your wife is to simply help her. Do you help her clear the dishes from the table after meals? Do you carry heavy loads of laundry up the stairs for her? Does she put the kids to bed alone every night? She shouldn't! Help her get them ready or better yet, take over a few nights a week and give her a chance to relax. Put your dirty laundry in the hamper instead of leaving it on the floor where you take it off. Those things sound simple, but trust me — they go a long way with your wife!

Gentlemen, the only thing necessary for you to want to have sex is the smallest piece of visual stimulus and a functioning reproductive system. Your wife was made differently, and before you resent how God created her, take a step back for one moment and appreciate that she is functioning just the way God intended. Your wife needs relationship in order to desire sex with you. This is a great blessing to your marriage because it forces you to stay connected with her in order to get your sexual needs met. If she didn't have that need for relationship, the two of you might very well drift apart without even realizing what's happening. Instead of feeling offended that you seem to have to pay a price for sex with your wife (in the form of errands, backrubs, daily showers, etc.), be thankful that God has built in her a deep need for connection that forces you both to come together.

What you actually do in the bedroom is totally dependent on what you decide together as a couple. Sex that is holy and pleasing to God is just like the love described in 1 Corinthians 13: It's patient and kind. It doesn't demand its own way. It's satisfying and is approved by both husband and wife. Don't pressure your spouse into sexual behavior that makes her feel uncomfortable. Discuss what you desire and mutually agree on your time together.

Would you eat the same lunch every day for the rest of your life? Of course not — how boring! Your sex life should be the same way. Variety is the spice of life and your sex life should be just as exciting. Instead of viewing sex as a means to the goal of ejaculation, slow down and enjoy exploring each other's bodies. Make the journey as wonderful as the destination.

You have an amazing amount of control over your married sex life. Ask God to show you how you can serve your wife and meet her needs. You'll probably be blessed with a lot more sex, but the payoff is even greater than that: You'll be working as partners with God to increase your love for each other and His creative power in your marriage!

JUST TELL ME WHAT TO DO

- ❑ What changes do you need to make in your personal hygiene to become more attractive to your wife?
- ❑ How can you become a better listener?
- ❑ What do you need to do to have more quality time with your wife? Stop right now and schedule a date night with her.

❑ In what little ways can you help your wife around the house? Choose one or two and start doing them today. And don't announce them to her like you are expecting a sexual payback! Just quietly start serving her and trust God for the reward.

❑ Take a few minutes to fill out the Marriage Assessment in Appendix 5. Discuss it on your next date night

5

It's More Than Being a Woman

I would never assume the role of a spokesperson for all women; however, hundreds of conversations with ladies of all ages and backgrounds have revealed a few common threads in the feminine sexual experience. I hope you'll benefit from my own personal experience as well as the opinions and insights I've gleaned from all those precious women who have shared their stories with me throughout the years.

It seems so long ago now, but I still remember being on the playground of my parochial school and first hearing what sex entailed. I was mortified! How in the world could a man's penis fit inside of me?! And *why* in the world would I want it to and possibly find it pleasurable? These feelings and trepidation stayed with me throughout adolescence and surfaced again when I was older and started contemplating marriage.

During my engagement to Bob, hormones escalated and eventually dominated those early thoughts. Instead of wondering how it would possibly work, I began dreaming of when it would finally happen! I was filled with such a deep desire to be with this person God had placed in my life, to be joined together both spiritually and physically. The longing erased all my fears and questions about sex. Even the negative things I sometimes heard about sexuality and marriage couldn't rob me of the anticipation I felt. I was head-over-heels in love and ready for my happily-ever-after!

We had a wonderful wedding night. Bob and I had the blessing of both being virgins with no preconceived ideas of what sex should be like. We weren't anxious at all that first night and our intimacy felt so perfectly natural, like we were meant to make love like this for the rest of our lives. And to my surprise, I *loved* the act of sex! It wasn't anything like I had heard on that playground so long ago or like girls had whispered about on the bus. I enjoyed the first time and couldn't wait until I had the chance to experience the ecstasy of an orgasm, which came with time as Bob and I learned more about pleasing each other.

If you had told me then that the years following would bring dramatic changes to my newfound sexuality, I don't think I would have believed it. But change is inevitable, and we walk through seasons of our life just as every generation has before us. Specifically, sexual desires and passions become different for women than what it appears for men. My friends and I laugh and shake our heads when we consider how simple the process is for men: they don't need to think about much more than sex, their penises and how much they love using them![1]

The honeymoon stage of our marriage was tremendous and we just took it for granted that it would remain that way indefinitely. It didn't occur to us to find ways to keep it fresh, exciting, important and fulfilling for both of us. Sex gradually became a mundane task for me. Bob is an achiever and I felt the

---

1   I certainly don't mean any disrespect to men; many of them have spent years becoming skilled lovers and are very considerate of their wife's needs. The fact remains, however, that women's bodies and hormones go through tremendous changes over the course of a lifetime and require much more attention and maintenance for a fulfilling sex life than men's do.

responsibility to help him pursue God's calling on his life. The cares and worries of our busy schedules choked out romance, serving each other, and honest communication about our individual needs and the needs of our marriage. I longed for something new to be excited and passionate about and returned to school to finish my college degree, thinking that might make a difference in our marriage. It did bring new things to talk about but also added to our time crunch and my stress.

We also decided to have children around this time, which was a wonderful experience but brought a whole new host of complications and strain. It was during this difficult time that Bob and I finally woke up to the reality of married sex: If we didn't make intentional choices to fan the flames of desire for each other, it was destined to flicker and eventually go out. Through many years of honest communication, prayer and being receptive to the promptings of the Holy Spirit, we reclaimed our early passion and once again started anticipating and enjoying lovemaking.

Every season of our lives together has brought changes to our minds, bodies and spirits that all have to be considered and reconsidered when we come together for intimacy. We'll look at some of those seasons next, and it's my hope that you'll find encouragement for whatever it is you happen to be walking through at this time.

WOMEN'S SEXUAL SEASONS

Sexual Education

Your sexual education started before you could walk or talk as you were held by those who raised you. Women who experienced good, loving relationships as they grew are blessed to have slowly learned about sexuality in a healthy environment. Unfortunately, many women are exposed to sexual abuse or neglect. These experiences can impact a woman's desire (or lack of it) throughout an entire lifetime. If you have issues stemming from your childhood, I urge you to find a qualified Christian counselor who can help you find healing through the power of the Holy Spirit.

Dating and/or Courting

Hormones are in overdrive during adolescence and young adulthood as women search for a partner and experience "falling in love." Any trepidation over intercourse is generally overridden by desire at this stage. Today's young people are waiting longer than ever to marry extending the season of dating and courtship. For many men and women, this results in multiple sexual experiences with a number of partners. Others struggling to maintain their purity may jump into a marriage too quickly, thinking they are honoring God by avoiding sexual temptation. Such quick decisions may bring regret in the future. While I don't believe there's one ideal time line for dating and choosing a mate, once you do find the person you want to marry, hormones make saying "Goodnight" more and more difficult. If you are single, I strongly suggest you find a godly mentor who will hold you accountable as you date and then get as much input as you can on your choice of a marriage partner. Ask everyone who knows you and loves you what they think of your choice! Do they see any potential problems? Are they concerned about any character flaws? It's wise to rely on others' objective opinions during this time when your hormones may be yelling louder than your brain!

Just Married

These early years of marriage can either be sexually blissful or somewhat confusing, depending on what expectations, beliefs and sexual knowledge a couple brings to the marriage bed. High desire and raging hormones generally continue to draw a couple together regardless of the quality of lovemaking. There is definitely a learning curve as husbands and wives continue to learn more about each other's bodies and needs. The passion of this stage is usually what couples long to recreate in later years.

Pregnancy and Babies

After delivery, many women experience painful intercourse for a matter of weeks and even months due to episiotomies, tearing or the stress of birth. I've found this to be a very common problem that can be remedied as long as a couple is patient and the husband in particular is tender. In addition to the physical challenges, new mothers may feel overwhelmed by the needs of a newborn. They may experience guilt over their inability to meet their husband's sexual needs at this time as well. Patience on the part of both partners is absolutely necessary as your marriage adjusts to this tiny newcomer. Just as you don't want your husband's career to distract him from your marriage, your husband doesn't want to lose you to your new career of "Mothering." Balance is the solution! Involve your spouse in caring for the baby and find ways to let him know that you are still madly, passionately, in love with him.

One last thought on this topic: Some couples make the mistake of thinking that having a baby will improve their marriage and/or sex life. This one for sure is not the answer! If your marriage needs a change, a baby *will* bring change! But it will also bring new challenges, new stress, new time constraints, and new frustrations.

Sexual Prime

Physiologically speaking, most women experience their sexual prime between 35 and 45 years of age. Of course, this season is impacted by factors other than your age; the intensity of your relationship and the satisfaction of your marriage are capable of either quenching your newfound desire or making it burn even hotter. Personally, these years were the most sexually fulfilling of my life. There were days I couldn't wait until the next time, and multiple orgasms weren't unusual. Your husband, of course, will absolutely love this season as well if he has a normal sexual appetite! If you are blessed to be walking through this season, do everything you can to make the most of it. Your sex life won't disappear in coming years, but why not enjoy this time when nature is working with you to make sex full of fireworks?!

Menopause

Women may start experiencing menopause at age 45 and up. I highly suggest you read the Is It Time for a Pause? Chapter to discover how simple a process this really can be. As your body starts to change it doesn't have to be the end of sex or the enjoyment of it; you will, however, have to listen to your body like never before and work with what you have. I've learned how to read my body's cues and can easily tell when I'm under additional stress by how my body reacts. I've learned not to expect more than I know my body can deliver sexually. As a result, I'm willing to cut back in other areas so Bob and I can experience the sexual relationship I desire (closeness) and he needs (release) to be mutually fulfilled and enjoy our relationship to the fullest. It's critical that you are both pursuing each other (The Hunt) during this season; use the ideas from this book to strengthen your marriage.

Regardless of the season you're in, one of the best things you can bring to your bedroom is a humble, willing heart that is ready to serve your spouse in love. If you have given sex a bad rap, it will be intolerable, a chore and unfulfilling. I urge you to reconsider. Sex is as much mental as it is physical, and if you're willing to approach it as a gift from God that bonds your hearts together, it will accomplish wonderful things in your marriage. I'll be honest: there are days that I don't feel emotionally interested or physically able — but I know if I "let myself" enjoy and participate, it ends up being pleasurable for both of us.

WOMEN'S COMMON SEXUAL CONCERNS

Body Image

Have you ever stood naked in a department store dressing room with twelve different bathing suits on the floor, none of which you'd ever be caught *dead* in?! I know many women who have! It's amazing that even the thinnest, most beautiful women in the world still have some part of their body to obsess about. For me, it's my stomach. I check it out from every possible angle to see if anything might have changed since the last time I looked in the mirror. What is it for you? Your hips? Small breasts? Cellulite? Your weight? Stretch marks? The truth is, you can let your body rule your thoughts, or you can make your thoughts rule your body. If what bothers you is something you absolutely can't change, it's time to let it go and focus on what you do have control over. If what displeases you is a result of your choices, the good news is you can make changes!

The most prevalent body image concern women in our society have today is their weight. There are many reasons women are overweight but the biggest one is destructive eating habits. Do you eat to live or live to eat? Are you in control or is your appetite? There are lots of healthy eating ideas in this book and I hope you'll start making positive choices. You don't have to be a size 4 to enjoy taking your clothes off in front of your husband; if you're a 14 and happy about it, enjoy your body and allow your husband to indulge in it as well!

Aging

I remember going camping with a friend in our late twenties and showering in this large communal women's shower room. The teenagers in there seemed so much more toned than we were — and we still in our twenties! Even with all I've learned since then, I'm not sure if I could walk into that shower naked again at this age. I actually weigh less than I did when I got married, but things aren't proportioned the same way, nor do they look the same. Some women really get stuck on the aging their body has experienced, but if you are in love this should never be an issue. It's an honor to be growing old with Bob and I'm so blessed by the assurance that he will remain faithful to me even into our old age. It's also a comfort to be reminded of Proverbs 31:30: "Charm is deceptive and beauty is fleeting, but a woman who fears the Lord is to be praised." Every woman, no matter how beautiful, will grow old eventually. The beauty in my heart is what Bob has grown to love and treasure even more than what I offer him with my body.

Breast Removal

My mom had her left breast removed during cancer treatment when I was in the 8th grade. She never complained about it but was simply grateful to be alive. Years ago, radical mastectomies resulted in a woman's body looking like a war zone, but my mother never seemed bothered by the scars. Other women find such surgeries to be incredibly traumatic. The good news is that there are so many more options for women today than were for my mother. Continuing reconstructive surgery is a possibility as well as therapy for cancer survivors. Find out what you can do to maintain your sense of sexual attractiveness and refuse to let cancer rob your marriage of its passion. I've seen couples walk through such challenges with amazing grace for each other because their love is based on more than appearances.

Hygiene

Few women stop to really consider that their vaginas are an excretory organ. We menstruate for many years and have normal discharges for even more. Our vaginas create natural lubrication to enable intercourse, resist chafing and facilitate conception. Like it or not, you are destined to be "damp" for one reason or another almost every day of your life!

Modern women have a huge advantage in controlling discharges. We can shower, bathe, wear panty liners and find some way to stay fresh in almost every situation. You should become intimately aware of your normal discharges — their color, consistency, even their smell. Discharges are a wonderful way to measure sexual health. The same is true of your menses: become aware of your cycle and you're better equipped to respond to your body's signals.

Menopause brings with it a whole new cycle of excretions. None of these have to hinder your sex life as long as you're willing to respond to them in appropriate ways. As you did before menopause, make an effort to present a clean and pleasing vagina to your spouse just as you offer a clean and pleasing body. Find out what turns your husband on and be willing to serve him by meeting those needs. They might include freshly-shaved legs, a quick teeth brushing before intimacy, or some deodorant and a spritz of his favorite perfume. (Of course, all men are different. If your husband likes to see you sweaty and grubby at the end of the day, by all means, accommodate him!)

THE GIVING AND TAKING OF SEX

Every healthy relationship is filled with giving and taking. Giving involves selflessly serving your husband and meeting his needs. Taking is humbly allowing your spouse to serve you. Neither is superior. When giving and taking are balanced the result is satisfied, fulfilled partners who are even more motivated to continue blessing each other. While giving and taking play a role in every aspect of married life, we'll discuss how they apply to our sexual relationship in particular.

Giving

Your husband is the most precious person in your life. Your kids may be gems, but they will eventually have a life of their own and you will remain married long after they've left the nest. If you don't take the time now to learn about your husband and build a strong relationship, you may find yourself married to a stranger when the kids leave for good. Now is the time to make an investment in your future together.

One very important gift you can give is your submission. Many women shudder at this word, believing it means making themselves a doormat to every whim and fancy of their husband. Nothing could be further from the truth. Submission may feel uncomfortable at first but its harvest is peace in your heart and home. Sexual submission means that you should be willing to consider your husband's sexual desires and do your best to fulfill them.[2] Have you taken the time to explore your husband's body, touching, kissing and caressing every part? You want to claim his heart and soul and one of the easiest ways to capture his love and attention is by also laying claim to every inch of his skin! Instead of being a disinterested sexual partner, show him you're involved and enjoying his touches. Look into his eyes as he ejaculates and share the rush of emotions that fill his whole being. You have the wonderful privilege of bringing him to this height of ecstasy and at these moments he is open and vulnerable to your love and influence. Enjoy the moment and welcome him back for more! After all, *you* are the woman he desires. What a wonderful honor!

Taking

"Taking" sounds like a selfish act, but it's simply allowing your husband to give to *you*. Many men have told us that the pinnacle of their lovemaking isn't their own orgasm — it's their *wife's* orgasm! If your husband is a considerate lover, he will delight in giving you pleasure and watching and feeling your body's

---

2   You should not submit to desires that are ungodly. If your husband requests a sexual act that you're unsure about, seek out a Christian counselor or ask to talk with your pastor about it.

responses. Your orgasm is a great compliment to him; they make him feel capable, useful, loved and desired. They also form a bond between both of you as you express your pleasure in a moment of extreme vulnerability. Bless your husband by allowing him to serve you in this way.

If you've never experienced an orgasm, I strongly urge you to have a candid talk with your husband and start pursuing one right away! You might read the Basic Training chapter together as a starting point.

TAKING THE LEAD

Every man would love for his wife to be the ringleader in the bedroom at least once in a while. It gets pretty discouraging when men feel they have to beg for sex. Instead of sending the message that sex is burdensome, find ways to let your husband know that you still desire him and him alone. Notes, text messages, cards, planning a surprise night away — these are all ways to keep things fresh and show him he turns you on. If you have to, mark days on your personal calendar that will be set aside so you can be the pursuer for a change. There's no need to announce it to him as he'll pick up on your cues soon enough and will enjoy the game immensely. Don't always use the same strategies but keep him guessing. When you find something he especially likes, don't do it so often it becomes a predictable habit. Make him proud to be the one guy in the group of men who doesn't complain that his wife isn't interested in sex anymore. He will love you even more for it!

Choose one or two from the following list and practice pursuing your husband this week:

> Call your husband at work. (Make sure you're not on speaker phone!) Tell him what sexy plans you have for the evening.

- Slip your husband a note at the dinner table to tell him you're not wearing panties.

- Greet him at the door wearing an apron. Just an apron!

- Run a ball of yarn all through the house. Make it go from room to room, through furniture, etc. Give him one end and tell him a surprise is waiting on the other. While he's searching, go to the other end and tie it around your finger. Take off all your clothes and hide in a closet until he finds you.

- Leave your clothing in a trail on the floor leading to your bedroom. Don't answer the door when he comes home, and let him follow the trail to find you in bed.

- Give him homemade sexy coupons for a birthday gift. ("This coupon is good for one full-body massage.")

- For Fathers' Day, meet him in the bedroom wearing the tie the kids got him as a gift….and nothing else.

- Play strip poker. Or strip Candy Land. Or strip Chutes and Ladders. Which game doesn't really matter!

- Put all of the candles you own in your bedroom and light them all before he goes up to bed. (Remember to disconnect the smoke alarm in your room first!)

- Ask him to come look at something in the laundry room. Make love during the spin cycle.

- Buy a provocative outfit you'd never wear in public and wear it just for him while you cook dinner and eat.

- Some evening, suggest he take a shower to relax or clean up. Then climb in with him. Consider wearing a white t-shirt.

- Have a picnic in front of the crackling fireplace with all the works: warm blanket, romantic music and YOU!

SPEAKING WORDS OF LIFE

I'm always disheartened to hear men and women speaking negatively about their spouse and marriage. After all, the power of life and death is in the tongue![3] Our words spring from the overflow of our hearts and our actions and attitudes always follow the direction we chart with our lips. When we speak negatively, things tend to get more negative. Conversely, when we use positive words that encourage and edify, we invite God's grace and blessing into our marriages. Let your husband catch you talking behind his back — saying *good and praiseworthy* things about him! Tell others how he blesses you, what a good father he is and what you most appreciate about him.

Hebrews 11:3 tells us that "God created the world by His word...." We too have the opportunity to create peace and love in our marriages, families and relationships with each word we utter.[4]

Matthew 9 tells the story of a woman who suffered for years from an issue of blood. In verse 21 she chose to speak with hope instead of discouragement, "I shall be restored to health." These words served to buoy her determination to touch Jesus and find healing from her affliction. I'm sure negative words would have robbed her of the desire to reach out for help, trapping her in a hopeless future. Thankfully, she chose to speak words of life and reality soon mirrored her speech. You also have the opportunity to choose life or death with the words you speak. I pray you'll choose life!

When the patriarch Jacob was about to die, he called his children together and blessed them. Genesis 49 recounts what he said to each son. In particular, he said something beautiful to

---

3   Proverbs 18:21
4   For more on the impact of our words, I highly recommend *Framing Your World with the Word of God* by Leroy Thompson and *Faith and Confession* by Charles Capps.

Joseph in verse 25: "...the Almighty blesses you...with blessings of the breast and womb." It's my hope that you will find joy in the privilege of being a woman, regardless of which season you're walking through or whatever changes and challenges you may be facing. God wants to bless you, your body, your marriage and your sex life!

JUST TELL ME WHAT TO DO:

❑ Think back to your own sexual education. Was it frightening? Neutral? Healthy? How did it affect your views about sex?

❑ What season are you presently in? What sexual struggles are you facing? Read through the discussion on that season and make whatever changes are necessary to help you enjoy your sexuality even more.

❑ Take a truthful assessment of your body image. What parts of your body do you dislike? What parts are you especially proud of? Find ways to play up the areas you like. Are there choices you can make that will impact the places you're not so fond of? (If not, determine to avoid obsessing over them!)

❑ Are you serving your husband sexually? Pursuing him in meaningful ways? Find two ways to flirt with him this week.

❑ Are you allowing your husband to give you pleasure on a regular basis? Remember that this is generally a huge turn on for most men. Allow him the pleasure of pleasuring you! If you have difficulty having an orgasm or have never experienced one, talk to him about pursuing it together.

❑ Choose one or two ideas and take the lead in an intimate time with your husband.

❑ Stop and consider what kind of words you're using when talking about your marriage. Ask God to help you speak words of life.

6
Let's Open Up

Most couples are pretty good at communicating about the kids' homework, the plumbing bill and when the dog was last let out. These topics are generally informational. Start discussing the budget, what church to attend, and who has gained more weight over the holidays and things start to heat up. Now delve into the most sensitive of marital subjects: sexual intimacy. It's amazing how many of us desire an incredibly intimate sexual relationship with our spouse and how very little we actually communicate about the topic. We'd all like to say we "feel at one" with our spouse sexually, but without communication that dream will never become a reality. As long as we remain silent about our feelings, needs, desires and fantasies, what happens in the bedroom will remain the same for the rest of our married lives.

Bob and I strongly believe sex should be one of the most-discussed parts of our marriage. Passionate, pleasurable sex doesn't happen accidentally; it's the result of open, honest, timely communication. Honest discussions become even more vital when one partner is suffering from health issues that interfere with normal sexual function. When a husband and wife talk openly about their sexual struggles and victories, their marriage becomes even more intimate and the world sees a shining testimony of God's creative presence within their home.

Genesis 1:28 clearly states God's plan for marriage: "God blessed them and said to them, 'Be fruitful and increase in number; fill the earth and subdue it.'" This plan hasn't changed, and we should take the covenant of marriage as seriously as God does. Every married couple has the opportunity to grow their love for each other and share His love with the world, and this starts in part by communicating who we are and what we desire in life and in the bedroom. It's time to bring pleasure to our spouses, ourselves, and to God through communication and the building of a passionate marriage.

Why is talking with your spouse about sex so difficult? Because, unlike a discussion of the plumbing bill which is simply an exchange of information, talking about sex requires a huge amount of vulnerability. Sometimes our spouse is the last person we want to admit our frailty to, especially if the relationship is struggling and such an admission might make us seem weak. (If it's too difficult to even imagine talking with your husband or wife about sexual issues, you might consider writing some thoughts and ideas down on paper.) Truthfully, it's hard for just about everyone to feel exposed, regardless of the state of our marriages. How we deal with this fear boils down to trust. Can we trust our partner to not take advantage of this vulnerability? Will they gently listen to our disappointments and desires or will they respond in anger and hostility? Trust is absolutely vital to free and full communication, especially when the topic is as fraught with tension and emotion as sex can be. Still, the only way you are going to understand each other's needs and desires is if you've established an easy rapport. Such communication is based on the firm belief that this person who shares your life is trustworthy and will handle your heart with tender care. When both partners approach their marriage with this goal, they build trust in each other and add years of greater happiness to the marriage.

Increased communication will not only benefit your sexual life together but all the other facets of your relationship as well.

Browse your local bookstore and you'll find shelves full of books on sex, sexual positions, sexual techniques, sexual mood makers, and etc. For all of the resources, you'd think people were doing nothing but talking about and having tons of mind-blowing, fulfilling sex! Our experience with couples has shown that this just isn't so. Generally speaking, couples continue having sex the way they started early in marriage. That is, even though the frequency may decrease, the technique (conditions leading to sex, foreplay, positions, etc.) doesn't change very much. Unless it's discussed and intentionally changed, you'll follow the same pattern for lovemaking 20 years from now that you did the last time you made love.

When Bob and I got married, we didn't talk about our sex life at all. What we were doing seemed to be working pretty well. No one had given us a bona fide sex talk before our wedding so we were real amateurs; the little we did know was learned from friends with more experience. I'm not sure if we were embarrassed by the subject or maybe we just didn't realize the need for discussion.

Somewhere along the way things stopped working so well. It wasn't that we weren't having any sex at all, but the sex we were having became routine, unexciting and less frequent — the On, In and Out kind of sex discussed in another chapter in this book. As other issues came to the forefront of our marriage, we slowly came to the realization that our sex life was suffering as well. During this time of some major distress we finally came to the conclusion: "We need to talk more about our sex life!" We decided to discuss our likes and dislikes and what we could do to make the whole experience mutually satisfying and a more fulfilling part of our marriage.

Not all of those early conversations were easy. There were pride and egos involved; neither of us wanted to make the other feel they were sexually inadequate, and it took some humility to hear that what used to work wasn't working anymore. The sexual pattern we had followed for years was getting old, and we needed to add a few new sparks into our life. Changing the routine of sex by making love at different times, places, and in different ways made us start anticipating those moments as we used to early in our marriage. We also became brave enough to open up to each other, sharing some of our secret fantasies and finding ways to work them into our lovemaking. The process took time and patience, but it was fun! We experienced heightened sexual pleasure and a new spark in our relationship.

As a woman, I discovered that the aging process had brought more changes to my body than a few laugh lines. What had worked for me before just wasn't able to produce satisfaction anymore, or it was still good but didn't last as long. It was such a relief to share these things with Bob and know that he was willing and able to respond to my changing body. I started doing lots of reading about sexuality, sorting through all kinds of books for those small nuggets of information that we could apply in our marriage. Some ideas we discussed at the dinner table to avoid any pressure in the bedroom; others we put into practice right then and there in our bedroom. ("I read about this today. Do you care if I try it?") Most of all, we worked hard to keep the mood light and our attitudes playful. Some things worked and others were a miserable flop that left us exhausted and laughing, but everything we talked about and tried was worth it! Remember, things won't change unless you *talk* about it.

One conclusion we've come to is that communication is even more vital when you're stressed. There will be times when one of you desires sex but has so much on your mind that your body will simply not cooperate. Clear communication and a good sense of humor will keep these moments from becoming frustrating and hurtful for either of you. Along the same lines, sometimes a stressful day makes intercourse physically uncomfortable for a woman. If you verbalize this to your husband, he can lovingly accommodate your stress by either waiting for another opportunity or tenderly ensuring that the experience is comfortable for you. You can always attempt having sex when you're stressed, but sometimes the best plan is to wait for a better time when it's sure to be more enjoyable for you both.

Loving, honest communication will keep you both on the same page. When sex is good it's an amazing blessing, and when it's bad — we've discovered that it's still pretty good! — as long as you strive to maintain a lighthearted attitude and sense of humor. Start talking and see what amazing new heights of passion and pleasure are waiting to be reached in your marriage.

JUST TELL ME WHAT TO DO:

❑ What pattern of sex did you start your marriage with? Are you still using it, and is it still working?

❑ Are there any sexual techniques you're tired of? Any that aren't working anymore? Are there new ones you'd like to try?

❑ Do you always have sex the same way at the same time in the same place? Discuss ways to make it new and exciting by changing some of the details.

❑ Have you experienced stressful periods when sex was difficult or impossible? Talk about the circumstances that caused those times. How can you better communicate when you're too stressed for sex or when you need your spouse to be extra considerate?

❑ Begin communicating about your sexual relationship. Recognize that it may seem uncomfortable at first but the benefits are worth it. Be sensitive to your spouse by truly listening and then working to meet their sexual needs.

❑ Try to come to mutual agreements, and if you can't, be willing to compromise. You might not be capable of fulfilling each other's fantasies right away, but by continuing to communicate and lovingly work together, your sexual life can be "the ultimate." Why not?

7

Not Tonight...
I'm Too Tired!

Deb and I were recently enjoying some quiet time on a Friday afternoon at one of our favorite local restaurants. Seated around us were at least five business people (both men and women) working diligently on their laptops while simultaneously operating cell phones and hand held computers. Now, I know the business world is all about scheduling appointments and productivity, but this was 3:30 on a beautiful Friday afternoon. I carefully observed everyone and they all looked *exhausted!*

People in western cultures live life in the fast lane at record-breaking speed. Everything is fast and disposable. The unfortunate by-product of this lifestyle is tired couples who end productive workdays with sexually unfulfilled nights. "Not tonight, dear," isn't just being uttered by women, either; I increasingly see men in my practice whose exhaustion plays a large role in their sexual issues. I have workshops for my patients every week in the office, and attendance always jumps through the roof when the topic includes anything to do with being tired or fatigued. Who's in the mood for lovemaking if they're always tired?

While I rarely allow myself to reach the point of exhaustion, Deb and I aren't immune to this phenomenon. I recently arrived home after a busy day. My body was tired, I felt uncomfortable and sweaty and all I wanted to do was sit down. Deb looked at me with a twinkle in her eye and said, "Do you want to do it?" I honestly didn't hear her but continued on with the conversation about how tired I was. Later on, after a short bike ride together, I got a second wind and was feeling a little frisky, but now *she* was winding down and starting her bedtime routine. She said, "Bob, didn't you hear me earlier? I wanted to do it and you were tired. You must not have heard me." Gentlemen, take my advice. When your wife asks, "Do you want to do it?"…just do it!

There are several causes of fatigue and one of the most common is over scheduling. There's only so much one person can accomplish in 24 hours' time, and having an unrealistic To Do List is not only physically tiring, it's also emotionally exhausting. Some men experience fatigue due to stressful jobs that rob them of their energy. Women who juggle the roles of employee, mother and housekeeper are easily exhausted, especially if their husbands aren't willing to step in and help with the house and children. Children are also experiencing the results of our fast-paced society. We've created a sports and activity frenzy in America that is churning out exhausted kids.

Exhaustion can also be caused by physical challenges. The role of the thyroid gland is discussed in detail in the Turning Up the Heat Chapter. If your hands and feet are cold and the lower temperatures of fall and winter weather really get you down, make sure you read the information on thyroid function. Still, there doesn't have to be any specific organ involvement like the thyroid or other glands being overworked — maybe *you* are just overworked!

Whether your fatigue is caused by over scheduling or physical maladies, the result is the same: tired husbands and wives who barely have enough energy at the end of the day to brush and floss their teeth, let alone meet in the bedroom for a sexual rendezvous. Lack of sexual intimacy seems like an easy thing to let slide, but the truth is, what happens in between the covers has an impact on the emotional force holding the whole family together. United, fulfilled, sexually satisfied Moms and Dads are empowered to lead united, fulfilled, emotionally satisfied families. Letting sex slide can be a costly mistake.

OVER SCHEDULING

Building a passionate marriage is impossible if you don't spend time with your spouse. Deb and I have discovered that we have to intentionally schedule time together or it just doesn't happen; we literally pull out our calendars and block out periods of personal time each week to enjoy each other's company. Sometimes we make plans and other times we just hang out and relax. Not every date has to include dinner and a show; some of the best times we've spent together have been hanging out in the quietness of our empty nest home or local coffee shop. Even spending time working on a project together at home can foster intimacy, and there's the added benefit of being near the bedroom if the urge strikes. (In fact, "projects" in the garage or basement can be a nice change in location if you're feeling adventurous!) Scheduling time like this may be a bit more challenging if you have children at home but we believe it's absolutely necessary for a passionate marriage.[1]

If you feel you don't have time to block out a few hours for your husband or wife each week, I'd urge you to take a second to look at your schedule. It's amazing the amount of time we spend doing what seems important while completely overlooking the urgent needs of our spouses. One of our biggest time stealers is technology; we're so widely available that products meant to serve

---

[1] We have friends who routinely swap babysitting with another couple on Friday evenings to ensure they get at least a couple of date nights every month.

our needs have become slave masters. It's amazing how many people I see constantly jumping whenever their cell phone rings, a text message arrives, or their e-mail inbox says, "You've got mail." When did we stop answering calls at *our* convenience instead of every time an electronic gadget beckons?! Today, with free nights, weekends, family plans, and in-network favorites, you can be available 24/7. On-line addictions like gambling, surfing the Web and chat rooms can become huge distractions from your spouse. If you want to have more sexual intimacy, those activities should be limited so your calendar can contain personal couple time. When you do have couple time, *turn your phone ringer off!*[2] Trust me; callers will leave a message if it's really that important.

If you're the kind of person who can get so involved in something that you don't realize the hours flying by, purchase a kitchen timer and set it before you start a task. It's a simple solution that will help you be accountable for your time. It may also result in a pleased spouse, some great sex, and a very large smile on your face!

I especially want to give you permission to say "No," when someone asks you to consider taking on a project. You have the right and the ability to do this without hurting anyone's feelings, as impossible as that sounds, and it's easier than you've ever imagined. Deb and I have learned to very graciously reply, "I can't say 'Yes,'" to requests we can't take on at the moment, which is simply a polite way of saying "No." You may want to practice saying this to yourself in the mirror until you've memorized the exact phrase. You don't have to offer any reasons why and you'll find that turning projects down gets easier and easier with time,

---

2   An exception to this, of course, would be when you leave your kids with a babysitter and need to be available in case of an emergency. The simple solution is to only answer calls coming from your home phone or wherever the babysitter and children happen to be while you're out.

especially if one of the rewards is more time with your spouse and greater levels of intimacy!

FEEDING YOUR BODY ENERGY

The human body is like a rechargeable battery: it functions for awhile but slowly loses energy. When output starts slowing down, you place the battery in a charger, plug it into the wall and "feed" it more juice. Your body functions the exact same way; if you don't take the time to stop, recharge, and feed your body energy-rich nutrients, output will slow and eventually come to a grinding halt.

Over the course of my patients' treatment we focus on a week's diet journal. I've looked over thousands of them and it's very evident that most people eat food for pleasure rather than the nutrients food contains. They consume foods which have been cultivated in mineral-depleted soil and eat anti-nutrients like sugar and artificial sweeteners which deplete the body of vital minerals and metals. Liver function becomes compromised and the body becomes mineral deficient, with symptoms of exhaustion, fatigue, headaches and food cravings. Diets full of sugar or trans fat foods lower sex hormone levels, zinc levels and put a damper on sexual activity. Unfortunately, at almost every business meeting, church committee and special gathering the table is heaped with pastries, cookies and donuts. Still, patients who are overweight or have addictions to sugar, alcohol, or smoking often insist, "Dr. Bob, it's just in moderation!" These sincere folks are usually addicted to what they are trying to "moderately" consume while their habit is slowly robbing them of energy and damaging their quality of life and sexual pleasure. Determine to kill the sugar habit and you'll be amazed at how much more energy you'll have.

You should also start drinking water from a pure source. I don't suggest consuming well water (unless you have a reverse osmosis filter in your home) because it may contain toxic chemicals that have permeated the water table. I've treated patients who suffer from depression because of well water; toxic levels of manganese show up in their mineral tissue hair analysis. Some spring waters have the same problem, and municipal water out of the tap generally contains high levels of chlorine, which puts stress on the thyroid. Invest in a home reverse osmosis filter (generally the most cost effective method) or seek out a source of purified water. Many health food stores offer containers of pure water for pocket change, depending on the amount you purchase. And start carrying a bottle of water with you during the day as a reminder to drink more.

How much water should you be drinking? There are many theories about the recommended amount, but I normally tell people to drink a quart of water a day, which is sufficient for most people weighing less than 120 pounds. For a more customized number, you should consume one half ounce of water for every pound of flesh.[3] You should also take into consideration how many fruit and veggies you are eating as they contain water and can be figured into the equation. It's possible to drink too much water, which can deplete minerals, so you should not drink more than 100 ounces under normal circumstances.[4]

Any beverage which robs your body of minerals should be consumed minimally. Caffeine and caffeinated teas act as a natural diuretic. If you're a coffee drinker, limit the amount and use a combination of decaffeinated that is Organic Swiss water processed. Many companies use toxic chemicals to remove the caffeine, but this method of processing is natural. Deb and I

---

3   Using this calculation, a 150 pound person should consume at least 75 ounces of water daily.

4   Exceptions would include persons who sweat heavily perform physical labor, or those in extremely hot environments.

generally brew organic coffee with a blend of one quarter caffeinated and three quarters decaffeinated.

The caffeine found in coffee, sodas, high power energy drinks and over-the-counter pain remedies acts as a stimulant. Many of my patients suffering from insomnia consume some form of caffeine, which results in an overworked and congested liver. (A healthy, properly functioning liver is able to filter caffeine out of the system.)

For renewed energy, add minerals to your daily diet plan. A simple mineral source is Celtic Sea Salt ® (www.druglessdoctor.com). This isn't the same as standard conventional salt; it comes from the North of France and hasn't been tampered with like regular table salt. Conventional sodium chloride (Na/Cl), depending on the source, has aluminum and dextrose as an anti-caking ingredient. Aluminum is a potential factor in contracting Alzheimer's disease. I suggest using Celtic Sea Salt ® liberally. If you're concerned about salt's effects on blood pressure, only about 5 percent of high blood pressure cases are caused by salt intake. Your body needs the minerals found in this type of salt to act as the spark plugs in your system. Alfalfa tablets are also a very affordable way to get the minerals your body needs. I also encourage organic food because it's generally grown in mineral rich soil that hasn't been robbed of vital nutrients.

In the office or while consulting with clients I make use of a very simple test called the Zinc Taste Test.[5] I put a dropper full of zinc sulfate in a small cup and have my patients hold it in their mouths for ten or fifteen seconds before swallowing. If they don't taste the zinc (which should be quite bitter), this indicates they may have a zinc deficiency in their body. Most of my patients who are tired, depressed, in pain or exhausted taste nothing!

---

5   Available at www.druglessdoctor.com

Zinc is critical for many bodily functions, including insulin production. Insulin is necessary to deliver glucose to the cells, and glucose is the gasoline that keeps a body moving. Common symptoms of zinc deficiency include poor memory, slow healing, prostate enlargement and fatigue. Zinc can be depleted by eating wheat and soy products, so I encourage my patients to avoid eating both of these. It's fairly easy to switch to brown rice, spelt flour or other substitutes.

Every bite you put into your mouth has the potential to supply energy to your cells or rob them of energy. Start making healthy choices today!

PROPER BODY MAINTENANCE TO CREATE ENERGY

As contradictory as it sounds, regular exercise actually *increases* energy levels. Exercise increases blood flow, strengthens the heart muscle and promotes peaceful sleep. It also cleans out the lymphatic system, (the sewer system in your body) by moving lymph fluid. This system doesn't have a pump like the circulatory system does; it relies on the normal movement of your daily activities to push the lymph around. Increased movement during exercise literally pushes lymph fluid through the body more quickly, which keeps this disease-fighting system working at peak performance by eliminating toxins from the body.

Deb and I jog two miles every morning and then ride our bikes for three miles, even in the winter as weather permits. We work out three days a week with weights, bands, a mini trampoline and a Pilates routine. Find an exercise program that's challenging and enjoyable and a partner to help keep you motivated. You'll notice the benefits almost immediately!

Another necessary part of body maintenance to increase energy is correct alignment of the spine. As nerve pathways are kept open and clear, signals from the brain to organs and tissues are free to flow properly. Spinal alignment also maintains correct posture, allowing full expansion of the lungs and full oxygenation of all body tissues. More oxygen results in more energy! Regular massage is also very helpful to many of my patients. It helps keep muscles relaxed and reduces tension and spinal problems.

Proper sleep habits are absolutely mandatory in maintaining high energy levels. Most people need on average eight hours of restful sleep each night. Of course, this number varies from person to person. A truly rested person is able to go to sleep when they start to feel tired, sleep without waking through the night and wake up without the aid of an alarm clock, feeling rested and rejuvenated. You should allow your body to set your bed and wake times (as your job and family allow, of course). Cortisol levels are highest in the morning and are responsible for waking you up. They continue to drop during the day, eventually signaling you to go to sleep. You should rely on these hormonal cues to determine your sleep and waking times. For most people, this translates into a bedtime around 10pm. Plan your children's bedtimes early enough that you will still have some quiet time for lovemaking before the two of you get to bed. And don't confuse your body with artificial stimulants such as caffeine. The more you inhibit the natural cycle, the more you will pay the price in reduced energy, sleepless nights and unproductive, tired days. Consistent lack of sleep is a sure path to total burnout.

If you have difficulty falling asleep at night, you should limit computer and TV use in the hours before going to bed. Your mind needs time to wind down at the end of the day just as your body does, and the constant stimulation of television will keep this from occurring. You should also cover up all of the small lights on electronic devices before going to sleep, including the glowing numbers on your alarm clock. These may seem like insignificant sources of light but they irritate the pineal gland and can keep you from getting the deep, restful sleep your body needs.

Taking steps to increase your energy level will make you a happier more productive person. Having more energy also means increased interest in sex and the ability to follow through! The steps I've recommended have almost immediate benefits; you'll notice an increase in energy in just days as you resist over scheduling, feed your body energy-producing foods and nutrients and properly maintain your health. The payoff in your bedroom is just an added benefit of being an energetic, enthusiastic lover!

JUST TELL ME WHAT TO DO

❑ Take an honest assessment of your energy levels. Do you feel rested upon waking each morning? Do you have enough energy to fulfill daily tasks, or do you find yourself dragging through half of the day, longing for bedtime?

❑ Do you often decide not to be intimate in the evening because you simply don't have enough energy?

❑ Are you over scheduled? Are there activities that can be cut out of your schedule to afford more time for your marriage?

❑ Practice saying, "I can't say 'Yes,'" and do it routinely!

❑ Get out your calendars and schedule some personal time as a couple.

❑ Are you feeding your body food and nutrients that provide energy or drain energy?

❑ Are you drinking enough water?

❑ Commit to a regular exercise routine.

❑ Decide on a bedtime (for each member of your family) and stick to it!

❑ Commit as a couple to whatever steps are necessary for increasing your energy levels.

8

It's More Than On, In and Out

The longer I'm married, the more I realize how differently my wife and I are wired. I have a high libido and am relentless in my pursuit of her. She enjoys our sexual encounters but is not always as passionate about having sex; she's much more fervent about spending time together and sharing what's going on in our lives. Our experience with couples has proven this trend; women are much more concerned with the relational and romantic aspects of their marriage. In contrast, candid conversations with married men generally come to a vastly different conclusion: men's priorities are sex, food and recreation. Unfortunately, we've come to realize that most men are either in denial or ignorant to the fact that men and women differ physically and emotionally in their approach to sexuality.

Wives commonly express their frustration to us that they feel sexually rushed by their husbands, who move too quickly in their intimate time. Women need time to warm up, conversation, touching, caressing and foreplay, and too many of them walk away from sex unfulfilled because those requirements for orgasm are unmet. The media promotes this lopsided sexual experience with passionate — and completely unrealistic — love scenes full of fireworks, earthquakes and orgasms, all in the span of a few minutes! We've coined a phrase for this kind of sexual encounter: *On, In and Out!* Many women feel exactly this way:

their husband wants to get *on* them, get *in* them, and then get *out* and back to the next task. It's almost impossible for a woman to walk away from this kind of "lovemaking" with any satisfaction or the desire for more.

There are exceptions to this rule, and there are even couples where the wife is more interested in sex, but we have found the *On-In-and-Out* experience to be surprisingly common. So why do healthy men seem to always want to have sex? Well, it's possible for both men and women to *desire* sex, but only men *need* to have sex. This is a crucial difference between men and women, a fact very few people even recognize. But once you understand the physiological drives that make men pursue sex, it becomes a great blessing in the bedroom.

In every man's body there are two small glands called the "seminal vesicles." These glands have a profound affect on men's sexual desire and behavior, though most men aren't even aware of their existence or function. I learned about them while taking an anatomy class and actually dissected them in a cadaver. The seminal vesicles are probably the most neglected tissue discussed in human sexuality.

Each seminal vesicle looks like an overcooked, deflated hot dog. They're about four or five inches long and nestled inside each vesicle is a coiled tube that continuously creates seminal fluid. Since they never cease production, the seminal vesicle keeps filling up after each ejaculation. As they fill with seminal fluid, the vesicles swell and stretch out much like a coiled garden hose tends to stretch out when filled with water. The seminal vesicles can't release any of the seminal fluid other than by ejaculation, and when ejaculation doesn't occur for a prolonged period of time, the swelling of the vesicles can actually make a man's testicles ache. This may sound unusual to you ladies, especially because it sounds like an odd and ridiculous excuse to get you into bed, but it's true!

When the seminal vesicles are full of fluid, men have a few options to release the pressure. The most obvious is to initiate sex with his partner. If that doesn't happen, he may fantasize about other women while engaging in self-stimulation (masturbation). He may even experience ejaculation as a result of a sexual dream, fondly called a "wet dream." It's also not uncommon for a man to discover leakage of the seminal fluid in his underwear if the pressure isn't relieved by ejaculation.

This normal sexual process involves much more than your husband's genitals, however; it's closely connected to his largest sexual organ: his brain! Closely surrounding the seminal vesicle is a network of pressure-sensitive nerves called the "vesicle plexus." A plexus is a group of tightly-knit nerves with a specific function, and this particular group of nerves alerts the hypothalamus of the amount of pressure being placed on it by the swelling of the seminal vesicles via the information superhighway of the spinal cord. The hypothalamus, in turn, contains a unique structure of specialized "neural circuits" which are specifically designed to trigger sexual arousal in response to the messages received from the vesicle plexus. So as each seminal vesicle swells and presses against the vesicle plexus, a message is sent to the hypothalamus that essentially says, "Pressure's high! Start thinking about having some sex up there!"

The hypothalamus faithfully responds by stimulating the release of testosterone (by the testes and adrenal glands) into the blood stream. Testosterone is the sex hormone at work in both men and women's bodies that triggers a conscious awareness of sexual need.

A word on testosterone is in order. In my clinical practice, I've observed an epidemic of men who are unable to respond to the thought of sexual intimacy because they are simply over-worked, stressed, and eating too many toxic foods. In short, their endocrine system is exhausted! This is easily treated with a glandular tissue supplement and minerals to revitalize this essential part of the brain. If you are a man with no desire for sex it's not necessarily psychological, it may simply be that your body is overloaded and unable to function properly. There are other reasons for a diminished libido which are discussed in The Erectile Dysfunction Chapter, but a low-functioning hypothalamus is one that is often overlooked.

So if a man has recently ejaculated and his seminal vesicles are relatively empty, no pressure is placed on the vesicle plexus and no message is sent to the hypothalamus. No message, no dump of testosterone into the blood stream. No testosterone dump, no extreme awareness of sexual desire. However, if ejaculation hasn't occurred in a while and the vesicles are filled to bursting with fluid, vesicle plexus sends a message, the hypothalamus dumps out testosterone, and your average male turns into a panting, sexual beast! The knowledge of this wonderful system (isn't God an awesome Creator?!) should bring a sigh of relief to both men and women. No, your husband isn't a sex-crazed maniac, ladies; his healthy body is simply performing exactly the way God intended it to! The process explains why a man who recently had sex can go about his business focused and determined, while a man who has a large buildup of seminal fluid can't walk by a lingerie store without an intense spiritual battle for pure thoughts. The timing is unique for each man; some may go days before sufficient seminal buildup starts the process while others may go only hours. But once the proverbial dam breaks, a man's mind is sensitized to every sexual stimulus he comes across. Involuntarily, a man finds himself intensely and powerfully attracted by sexual thoughts and fantasies, including acute awareness of the women in his immediate vicinity. As a result of this purely biological function, men are subject throughout their adult lives to the compellingly distractive and recurrent sexual cycle of involuntary arousal, bodily excitation and ejaculation followed by temporary serenity.

This is by no means an excuse for immorality or callous treatment of women. Ladies, if your husband ever tries to use this biological system as justification for brutish and selfish demands, you have my full permission to get out this book and hit him with it! But this knowledge *does* give wives the wonderful opportunity to understand their husband's sexual needs and drives and to help them cope with distracting sexual impulses by offering a warm and welcoming sexual outlet in the marriage bed.

This isn't to say there's not a place for *On-In-and-Out* sex within marriage. There are occasions in our routine when Deb is not so interested in sex but she recognizes that I have a dire need for release. Because we're honest and open in our communication, I can express that need to her without fear that she'll roll her eyes and label me a "sex maniac." And because she realizes that not every sexual encounter has to include fireworks and earthquake orgasms, she willingly and lovingly allows me an *On-In-and-Out* experience. (Some of you may call this a "Quickie.") She also knows that I am much easier to get along with when I've had that sexual release. We both gain spiritually from the experience as well. Deb is blessed for serving me sexually, and my heart is drawn to hers in thankfulness for her selfless giving. She also provides me the wonderful gift of a suppressed libido for a time, and the bombardment of sexual stimuli is easier to combat after that pressure has been released. Everybody wins!

Husbands, a word of advice. Your wife will be much more willing to engage in healthy *On-In-and-Out* sex if she knows that in the near future you will take the time to have a prolonged sexual encounter with her that includes tender caresses, loving conversation, lots of foreplay and a focus on her sexual fulfillment. If all of your sex is the down-and-out, over-in-three-minutes kind, expect her to grow more and more resentful and less and less willing to consider your swelling seminal vesicles over time!

Timing is incredibly important when it comes to the two of you coming together in a mutually satisfying sexual rendezvous. And women aren't exempt from timing, as you know if you've ever dealt with a wife suffering from premenstrual syndrome![1] Shortly after finishing menstruation a women's hormone level peaks. This is in preparation for ovulation, when a woman is at her most fertile for 24-48 hours. It makes sense, then, that God designed women to be more sexually aware at this time in their cycle. Husbands, you would be wise to become very informed about your wife's menstrual cycles, because it will greatly benefit you in the bedroom! A few days after her period ends is the time to initiate long, intimate lovemaking sessions; it's when she's most physically and emotionally responsive and most likely to achieve an orgasm. Following ovulation (which generally occurs about 14 days after her period starts), the sex hormones decline to prepare for menstruation if there's no fertilization and pregnancy. These few weeks after ovulation are generally marked by declining sexual interest, and it's when she will probably be relieved if you understand that she's not so willing to jump through sexual hoops. She may be experiencing the preparation for menstruation with its mood swings, bloating, etc., which understandably doesn't make her feel very sexually appealing or adventurous. This is the time for gently requesting *On-In-and-Out* intimacy. You might approach her by saying, "I know you're not feeling very sexual right now, but I would love to just be with you and enjoy some sexual release. I want to direct my desires toward *you* and not feel so overwhelmed by other stimuli. Would you consider meeting that need for me?" Trust

---

1 Women who have had a total hysterectomy or are in menopause may still have a hormonal cycle even if they have stopped menstruating.

me, husbands, your wife will be astounded by your gentleness and consideration as well as touched by your vulnerability and desire for godly thoughts. And if she isn't? Ask God to speak to her heart and keep on trying!

If you are struggling to maintain sexually pure thoughts, there are a few things you can do to be successful. First of all, hide the Word of God in your heart. A good verse to memorize is Psalm 119:9 and 11. "How can a young man keep his way pure? By living according to your Word. I have hidden your Word in my heart so I will not sin against you." The Holy Spirit can help you control your sexual desire and reserve this sacred act for your spouse alone.

Now that you realize how important timing is for a mutually fulfilling sexual experience, it makes sense to put some thought into *when* you should have sex. Plan to have sex?! Absolutely! Although occasionally sex will occur spontaneously, the demands of work, family and friends prevent those thrilling surprises from happening very often. A smart couple will intentionally carve out time to spend together which may or may not include sex. For example, (in our early marriage and child rearing) when I'm on the road for a few days, I often purchase flowers or a small gift for Deb. If Deb is out of town, I'll welcome her home with romantic music playing, candles in our bedroom, and possibly even some homemade whipped cream. Deb does the same for me, occasionally purchasing lingerie and preparing in ways she knows will really turn me on. What a wonderful way to reconnect after an absence!

It actually seems crazy *not* to plan for sex. I see business travelers at airports who are totally drained and patients at my practice who are worn out. I see couples who work shifts and barely see each other or who work multiple jobs to make ends meet. If they aren't planning for intimate time together, I can almost guarantee it isn't happening. The plans don't always have to include sex, either, although time spent focusing on each other usually leads to physical intimacy. Even if it doesn't, your relationship will be strengthened and the loving feelings that are developed will certainly increase the odds for sex in the future. All of this planning is really nothing more than dating your spouse. Don't let being married stop you from dating each other! Your plans can be as simple as a walk, a bike ride, or a picnic.

I'll never forget a date I had with Deb while traveling in Florida. I had done my planning — I took massage oil, candles, and a CD with her favorite music. We had very intense whole-body sex without the stress of work and children. When we're attending business seminars, we take time to have spontaneous sex in the hotel room. These planned times of intimacy have truly been one of our secret weapons as a couple and have kept our marriage amazingly passionate. They'll do the same for you!

Gentlemen, now that you realize how incredibly different men and women are sexually, let me offer some specific suggestions that will greatly improve your sex lives. I'm addressing men here because, generally speaking, we're the ones who want more sex. If you're a woman who happens to have a higher libido than your husband, these should be helpful to you as well. An important concept to remember is that *where your mind goes your energy flows.* Simply put, if you desire more sex, you should be devoting energy in the pursuit of that goal! Sometimes I talk with men who are experiencing marital challenges, yet they're so busy scheduling a golf game or a hunting trip that it's almost inevitable they aren't having any sex with their wives. Many men don't consider romancing their wives or creating the emotional and physical intimacy that will almost guarantee them a sexual interlude. You may still get your wife in bed with this kind of thinking, but to have an absolutely wonderful sex life you need to include your *wife* in your day planner and consider the times that *she* might want to be intimate, not just the times that *you* want sex. This may be the most important marital lesson you can learn; your wife, believe it or not, desires and wants your companionship, love, support and your time. When those needs are met, she will almost assuredly also want sex!

First, devote time to quality conversation and tender moments together. Happy marriages are based on deep friendship. Isn't it uncomfortable when you're with a couple who obviously aren't friends, but enemies? When friends become unfriendly, we walk away from the friendship, yet too many spouses treat each other terribly and then wonder why their relationship suffers. If you wouldn't make sarcastic remarks to a friend, you certainly shouldn't be making them to your spouse. If you wouldn't put down a friend in front of a crowd, you shouldn't do it to your spouse, either. In fact, building your spouse up in front of other people makes a huge statement to your spouse — and the crowd — about how much you value them. The words you speak will build your house or tear it down, so consider them carefully![2] For the same reason, don't hang around people who consistently speak negatively about their spouses. Sometimes when a same-sex group gets together they spend much of their time putting down the opposite sex. This only leads to dissatisfaction, and to be honest, it's sinful! Be the brave person who redirects the conversation toward something edifying about your spouse; it will bring gentle conviction to the others and they'll admire you for it. It will also bless your spouse when they hear that you've been talking about them (good things!) behind their back.

---

2   "Each of you should be slow to speak, quick to listen, and slow to become angry." James 1:19

Secondly, spend more time in the Word, exalting and praising God, and asking the Lord to speak to you. When you're in your prayer closet, take time to be quiet and listen to His Spirit. Allow Him to be your Guide in your intimate relationship with your spouse. After all, the Creator of the whole thing should know how to best make it work! He promises to guide us into all truth, which includes understanding what your spouse desires, how to become better friends, and even subjects you might need to discuss. Some of our most intimate moments have followed discussions about what the Holy Spirit is revealing to us about our marriage.

Husbands, start to become a pursuer of your *wife* instead of just a pursuer of sex. This means that meeting *her* sexual needs should become as important to you as meeting *your* sexual needs. This comes naturally for many men who get enormous emotional satisfaction from stimulating their wives and sharing their climax. Other men haven't yet realized that half of the pleasure of sex is enjoying their partner's orgasm as much as their own! Sadly, many women have never achieved orgasm, and it's somewhat stunning that they still desire intimacy at all. Husbands — trust me! — it's not only in your best interest to put a smile on her face, it's also biblical! 1Corinthians 7:3 states, "The husband should give to his wife her conjugal rights, goodwill, kindness and what is due her as his wife...." If you're unsure about what she needs, bring it up in a quiet moment and let her know that you are willing to learn. This could mean swallowing your pride, but the payoff in intimacy will be worth it. Remember that what she tells you may include what *not* to do as much as what she does enjoy. Don't pressure her to perform, but reassure her that this is something you're willing to work on when she's in the mood. Take your time and enjoy learning how to be a considerate lover.

And while we're talking about meeting her needs, it would be in your best interest to start doing those extra little chores around the house that would take stress off your wife. Until her "To Do List" is finished in the evening, sex is just another task on the list! Ask her what you can do to help. Offer to put the children to bed so she has time for a bath. When men tell me they're dissatisfied with their sex lives, I ask a few questions right off the bat: Do you empty the dish washer? Pick up after yourself? Lower the toilet seat? Squeeze the toothpaste at the end? Help with dinner? Don't be resentful, feeling you are "paying" for sex with your wife. No, you are investing in a relationship that gives huge dividends when properly cared for!

Some of you are in a difficult position, desiring changes in your sex life when your spouse doesn't seem to care. Please be encouraged! We've seen one partner start making changes in their health and their approach to sex, and the disinterested spouse slowly wakes up as they see positive results. Couples like this often become partners in improving their relationship, which is God's plan from the start! Determine that you will make wise and godly choices despite what your spouse does or doesn't do, and give God time to work in their heart as well.

We just read an e-mail from a woman who receives our correspondence and is familiar with the work we're doing on the subject of sex and romance. She was excited to inform us that she had recently been communicating with her husband about what he could do to please her sexually. Her husband often rushed through sex and she had never expressed wanting anything different. After a few honest discussions, he became an expert at pleasing her and they are enjoying the best sex of their 35-year marriage! Every couple can improve upon the wonderful blessing of sexuality. It's our prayer that your marriage bed will be filled with honesty, tenderness, and joy!

JUST TELL ME WHAT TO DO

❏ Reserve some quiet time to candidly discuss your libidos. Whose is higher/lower? How do you feel about the frequency of your lovemaking? Do you need to make adjustments to satisfy the needs of your partner?

❏ How often is your lovemaking slow and tender, and how often is it the On, In and Out kind? How do you feel about these percentages? (Remember that On, In and Out sex has a place in your marriage as long as you both feel satisfied by its frequency.)

❏ What changes can be made to ensure mutually satisfying intimacy as often as each partner desires it, and On, In and Out sex as often as each partner is agreeable?

❏ Do you have times of intimacy that are slow, tender and mutually satisfying?

❏ If you're a woman, are you achieving an orgasm during sexual encounters? Are you graciously communicating how your spouse can help you reach orgasm? If you're a man, are you willing to humbly listen to your wife's requests and help her in this capacity?

❏ What are some common reasons that you turn down sex? Are there things your spouse can do to make you more willing to have sex?

❏ Are you intentionally planning times for intimacy, whether or not they include lovemaking?

9

Created to Create

The first few chapters of Genesis give incredible insight into God's vision and values. Almost everything we need to function as His children is provided at little more than a glance. It quickly becomes evident that God holds in the highest regard his relationship with his children and their relationships with each other. We marvel at the creation of man, the determination that man should not be alone, the creation of woman, and the institution of marriage. All of this by the second chapter!

Genesis 1: 27 states, "So God created man in His own image, in the image and likeness of God He created him; male and female He created them."[1] It's amazing to consider that our creative God would bless us with the ability to create ourselves. And yet we do — and with great joy. From finger-painted smears on the walls to portraits on the ceiling of the Sistine Chapel; from chopsticks on the old upright piano to Beethoven's Fifth Symphony, we create from the cradle to the grave. And not only did God gift us to create, but in His likeness we are blessed with amazing imaginations which churn out masterpieces that express our every emotion. Yes, our Creator in His wisdom made each of us a creator in our own small sphere of influence.

---

1   All Scripture is from the Amplified Version unless otherwise noted.

Within marriage, our creative power explodes. In the very next verse, God blesses the man and woman, saying, "Be fruitful, multiply, and fill the earth, and subdue it (using all its vast resources in the service of God and man); and have dominion over the fish of the sea, the birds of the air, and over every living creature that moves upon the earth." This verse states our purpose: to procreate both physically and spiritually, in the sexual act of procreation to populate the earth and provide a larger family to enjoy fellowship with God and with nature, and spiritually as we partner with God to fulfill His purpose and destiny for mankind.

Our marriage relationships have incredible creative power when we walk in unity as a couple. As husband and wife share a common purpose, there is little they cannot accomplish together. This was God's intention for marriage from the beginning; His plan was for the Garden of Eden to be established throughout the whole world as Adam and Eve lived in harmony and expressed their creative imaginations together.

A marriage based on godly values and purposes has unbelievable creative power. Matthew 18:20 states, "Where two or three of you are gathered together in My name, there I am in the midst of you." Marital intimacy (sexual and spiritual) actually invites God's presence into our midst. This partnership between a husband, wife and God first results in a new dimension of unity, creativity and power, further igniting the passion and joy within the marriage relationship. The holy union of three then turns their attention outward, creatively impacting the world for Christ. God's empowerment in a couple fully submitted to Him and each other is destined to attract attention, drawing others to a saving knowledge of Him.

In a traditional wedding ceremony the officiating pastor pronounces that a man and woman are husband and wife together. That statement is followed by a very serious charge from heaven itself. "What therefore God has joined together, let not man put asunder." The unfortunate truth is that divorce rates in the church mirror those of the secular world. The awesome creative potential of many Christian marriages is snuffed out by divorce, and even if couples remain married, the creative power of marriage is severely limited as they tend their wounded relationship rather than focusing on building God's kingdom.

God intends for married couples to bring this creative power to the world. Healthy marriages result in much more than happy couples; they bring life and vitality to children, homes, churches and communities. God is very passionate about the creative power of marital intimacy. Genesis 38:9-10 states "…but Onan knew that the family would not be his, so when he cohabitated with his brother's widow, he prevented conception, lest he should raise up a child for his brother. And the thing which he did displeased the Lord; therefore He slew him also." Many Bible translations read, "…and he let his seed drop to the ground." Onan deliberately thwarted the creative power God intended for the sexual act and denied his brother's widow any children. In effect, he wasted the seed that God intended to bless with life. And God is interested in seed! It is the method He has chosen to give his children great creative power in their most intimate act of love.

When we are following Christ wholeheartedly, our personal relationships abound with energy, ideas, love, passion, tenderness, vision, like-mindedness, and peace. As relationships deepen, so should the blessings that flow from them. Imagine then what is possible from the most intimate relationship between a man and woman. The creative power unleashed by the spiritual, emotional and sexual unity of a marriage provides almost limitless resources for both husband and wife. We have found this to be true in our own relationship. People commonly ask us, "Where do you get your energy?" or, "How do you get ideas so fast?" The simple answer is that the unity of our marriage welcomes the presence of the Holy Spirit in our lives, and the result is creative power that spills over into every aspect of who we are: spouses, parents, business owners, health practitioners, and friends. We praise the Lord that this has enabled us to help countless others as they walk alongside us on this incredible journey toward eternity.

Creating a marriage that flourishes with the creative power of God's presence takes time. As you juggle children, careers, family, and life in general, remember to reserve enough time and energy to take care of each other's needs. Some days this will mean being sexually intimate, but other times it will be a listening ear or a shared opinion or some simple encouragement. As you partner with God and each other, your marriage will grow in intimacy and creative power as He intended!

JUST TELL ME WHAT TO DO

❑ Thank God for the gift of creative power in your marriage.

❑ Take an honest assessment of your marriage. Is your focus inward due to struggles and conflict? Ask God to bring healing to those areas that keep you focused within.

❑ Are there ways your marriage is impacting those around you? Ask God to join your partnership and show you ways the creative power in your marriage can reach out to a world in need.

10
Ladies: Sex is an
Inside Job

L adies, imagine you're getting ready for an exciting night out. You choose your sexiest outfit, take extra time putting on your makeup and mist on your favorite perfume. You're all ready to go out — and still not in the least bit interested in having sex with your husband. (Ironically, it's exactly those special touches that start your husband's sexual engine!) Sound familiar? It probably does to many of you and we're not a bit surprised, because sex and sexiness start on the *inside* and then work their way *out*. If you're not feeling sexual or sexy, no amount of clothing, makeup or perfume is going to flip your switch to "On!" If your body isn't functioning properly at a cellular level, your sexuality will eventually be affected.

I treat many common sexual problems in my practice which originate at the cellular level, and I'm glad to tell you that almost all of them can be treated naturally without the use of medication. Following is a list of the symptoms I most commonly assess in my female patients. We'll discuss how to treat each one by focusing on inside-out restoration. Internal health improvements bring about external changes in sexual function.

Common Female Sexual Challenges

➤ Tender breasts with or without a heavy/persistent menstrual flow

➤ Chronic vaginal yeast overgrowth

➤ Pelvic and spinal pain

➤ Painful penetration due to vaginal dryness

➤ Painful penetration due to constipation

➤ Lack of desire for intimacy

➤ Poor self image

TENDER BREASTS AND A HEAVY OR PERSISTENT MENSTRUAL FLOW

Tender breasts and a heavy or persistent menstrual flow are commonly seen in women experiencing estrogen saturation or dominance in their bodies. Estrogen promotes growth within cells and is normally elevated at the beginning of the menstrual cycle, but it's balanced by another steroid hormone called progesterone, which peaks a bit later in the cycle during ovulation. The balance of these two hormones is critical. The causes of estrogen dominance include:

An overabundance of synthetic estrogens may be found in the water supplies of many municipalities. The source of estrogen in drinking water may be human hormone replacement/birth control pills or estrogen that is fed to animals raised for meat.

Synthetic hormones (xenhormones) are found in common household items including plastics.[1] These plastics are also used as a coating on the inside of cans. The cans which are heated to prevent contamination are then filled at the manufacturing plant;

---

1   Included are Number 7 recyclable containers.

the estrogen is released in minute but accumulative amounts. This is discussed further in the Liver Detoxification Chapter.

I don't encourage soy products of any kind to any of my patients, whether male *or* female. Soy raises estrogen levels, depletes the body of zinc, and minimizes trypsin, an important enzyme beneficial in fighting cancer. [2] Presently, soy is often produced from genetically modified seeds and then heated to high temperatures, which renders it very low in any active nutritional value.

The estrogen/progesterone balance can once again be brought under control by promoting optimal liver function. I would encourage you and your spouse to eat Dr. Bob's A-B-C's daily:

A. one-half of a red apple

B. one-third cup of organic beets, either raw and grated or baked[3]

C. four or five organic baby carrots or one medium carrot

These three items will help your liver process the environmental toxins from your body, and proper liver function will help balance estrogen and progesterone levels.

I also encourage my patients to take a whole food B vitamin every day. B vitamins are required to process estrogen through the liver. Whole grain brown rice is a good source of B vitamins and can be eaten on your salad or sautéed with onions and olive oil. B vitamins are also produced in your colon; if you've been on an antibiotic within the past year, you should start taking a quality pro-biotic to re-establish the flora in your digestive tract.

---

2   Increased estrogen levels in men may lead to prostate difficulties.
3   See Appendix 2 for beet recipies.

Finally, my experience has shown that all women can take up to twelve milligrams of organic iodine a day and may do so indefinitely. (Japanese women have been consuming this amount safely for years.) Iodine assists the ovaries in making enough progesterone to balance estrogen; it also has been shown to reduce cystic breast disease.[4] An iodine program should be started slowly because it will cause halide compounds to be flushed from the body (see Turning up the Heat Chapter). While this will improve your health in the long run, the sudden flushing from the system may cause a metallic taste in the mouth, headaches, skin rash and possibly diarrhea or flu-like symptoms. These are all common signs that toxins are being released, especially bromine and chlorine. To ease the introduction of iodine, I suggest the following start-up program:

Week	Iodine Amount	Dose Per Day
1	3 mg tablet	1
2	3 mg tablet	2
3	3 mg tablet	3
4 and on	3 mg tablet	4

CHRONIC VAGINAL YEAST OVERGROWTH

Deb and I have been blessed by never having to contend with a yeast infection, but I've learned from many patients that these chronic infections can be a long-term nightmare that greatly interferes with sexuality. After treating many women who struggle with chronic yeast and fungus challenges I've concluded that **patients who have yeast and fungus infestations are normally addicted to carbohydrates.** That's probably an understatement; these ladies *love* sugar and refined grain products — pastries,

---

4   See David Brownstein's book, *Iodine: What You Need To Know About It.*

cookies, dried fruits, candy and chocolate, just to name a few. These high carbohydrate diets cause a huge burden of stress on the immune system, decreasing its ability to seek out and destroy fungus, bacteria and viruses.[5] The paralyzed immune system creates an environment that freely allows unfriendly bacteria, yeast and viruses to multiply. You will quickly experience these commons symptoms when your body is compromised: pain, fever, a cough, runny nose, etc. If you see a physician, they'll most likely treat the infection with antibiotics, which seek and destroy nearly every living "flora" organism in your body, including the "good" bacteria. Yeast and fungus are long-term survivors and are designed to resist the attack, so you're now left with a full-blown yeast infection and even *less* resistance due to decreased "good" flora bacteria! Your doctor will most likely prescribe an anti-fungal medication which controls your dilemma for a while — until you stop taking it. Once you go off it the whole vicious cycle starts over again. This process can go on for years, and for some ladies a whole lifetime. It's no surprise that yeast infections are a huge impediment to a mutually fulfilling sex life!

Women aren't the only partners impacted by these infections. It's possible for yeast from a women's vagina to pass into her husband's penis during intercourse, especially if he is also consuming a diet high in carbohydrates. Yeast can grow in his prostate and other reproductive tissues, causing possible pain in the groin, incomplete voiding of urine and discomfort during intercourse. The cycle may continue as partners continually re-infect each other.

---

5   See *The Wellness Book* by Herbert Benson, MD and Eileen M. Stuart, RN, MS.

As a result of these infections, both men and women may experience athlete's foot, finger- and toenail fungus, a coated tongue or yeast overgrowth in the ears. Some of my female patients have had secretions from their breasts and major yeast growth around their rectum and vagina. I've even seen patients who resorted to having their toenails removed because the fungus would not abate even with high power antibiotic and anti-fungal/yeast medications. The yeast fungus challenge is an inside out imbalance

You can perform a simple saliva procedure in your home which helps you preliminarily establish whether you have a yeast or fungus overgrowth. Upon waking in the morning, gather all the sputum (spit) that's in your mouth and release it into a cold glass of water; after a few moments, look to see where the saliva has gathered. The sputum should float on top of the water; if it sinks to the bottom this is a possible initial sign you may have a yeast and fungus issue. I recommend you consult a natural healthcare provider who may suggest further testing including nutritional microscopy evaluation or stool and saliva samplings.

When I treat patients with yeast overgrowth I use Gymnema (an herb which diminishes the taste for sugar) and chromium (an element) which eliminates the desire for sugar. We may also use a citric seed extract to control the yeast naturally. We use a product called Agrisept-L created from grapefruit, tangerine and lemon seed extracts. This product should be started slowly to avoid a massive flushing of destroyed yeast debris which can lead to flu-like symptoms. My patients start by taking three or four drops of Agrisept-L in four to eight ounces of water once a day for a week or two; then they take the same dosage twice a day for the rest of their treatment. I've taken ten drops of Agrisept-L for ten years as a preventative maintenance program. I also start my patients on a pro-biotic to re-establish healthy flora.

One of the most important methods of treating yeast overgrowth is establishing a life-long healthy eating plan. Foods should be consumed from the mid-glycemic range (from 55-80) on the glycemic chart Appendix 1.

PELVIC AND SPINAL PAIN

Have you ever seen a car driving down the road that looked like it was moving at an angle? Your eyes aren't playing tricks on you! The slang term for this lack of alignment is "dog tracking." When cars are exposed to the repeated jarring that comes from hitting potholes, speed bumps and ruts, the frame goes out of alignment. Over time, this misalignment causes the tires to wear out unevenly and at a faster rate. The mechanisms at the front of the car's stabilization bars may experience rapid breakdown. Car manufacturers know that proper alignment is critical for the long-term performance of the vehicle; that's why they suggest having the front end aligned at regular intervals.

I see patients in my office every day that move just like those unfortunate crooked cars! The most common reasons for spinal misalignment are poor posture, poor sleeping habits, stress, injuries from motor vehicle accidents, sports and exercise trauma, poor quality nutrition, and even the birthing process. Unfortunately, most people have not taken the time to have their spines checked by a skilled spinal specialist.

Many women walk around every day completely unaware that they have a misaligned pelvis and lower spinal vertebra. These misalignments are called subluxations, they can cause pain and inhibit nerve flow information from the brain. These symptoms frequently interfere with satisfying sexual intimacy. Spinal correction has given many women relief from menstrual cramps and groin pain. Because the uterus, bladder, vagina, rectum and ovaries are suspended in a woman's pelvis by muscles, ligaments and connective tissue which connect to the skeleton, the positioning of the spine and pelvic structure have a direct impact on the internal organs' ability to function optimally. Many women's sexual experiences are enhanced when the structures supporting their female reproductive organs are in their correct positions.

If you experience back pain during intercourse, I strongly suggest you have your spine checked. After chiropractic care, many women discover they are able to enjoy new sexual positions that were previously uncomfortable. Different lovemaking positions not only keep sex fresh and exciting, they also provoke different sensations for both partners.

PAINFUL PENETRATION DUE TO VAGINAL DRYNESS

While a man's penis may contribute a very small amount of lubrication in the form of seminal fluid during initial penetration, it's not nearly enough to prevent chafing and irritation during the entire lovemaking session. The vast amount of lubrication needed for sexual intercourse is provided by a woman's vagina. At least that's how God intended it! Unfortunately, vaginal dryness is a common complaint among women.

The pharmaceutical industry spends billions of dollars annually lulling consumers into the belief that the only way they are going to enjoy sexual intimacy is with a vaginal lubricant. Nothing could be farther from the truth! Adrenal health is a key to proper vaginal lubrication. Following a healthy diet and decreasing stress are simple ways to ensure a properly functioning endocrine system. As the sympathetic nervous system creates less stress on the parasympathetic nervous system, the mucous membranes throughout the body are kept supple and moist, including those in the vagina. See the Adrenal Gland Chapter for more detail on this important system.

For you ladies approaching or experiencing menopause, a lack of estrogen may affect your vaginal lubrication but adrenal gland health still plays a vital role during this season of life. I recently spoke with a woman who is fifty-nine years old. She's employed by a wellness health care facility and understands natural healthcare. She told me that her sex life is better now than ever since menopause. Please don't assume that menopause has to be accompanied by a dry vagina and fading sex life!

Young women aren't immune from vaginal dryness, either. Adrenal gland function has an extremely significant role in the creation of lubrication needed for intercourse regardless of one's age. Recently, a vivacious twenty-two-year-old, newly married woman attended one of our talks about sexual dysfunction. She had driven two hours to hear us speak and confided in us later that she often experienced vaginal dryness and did not enjoy sex. Instead of the typical blushing newlywed, she was dreading a marriage filled with sexual frustration that she felt would inevitably lead to divorce. After hearing our talk on adrenal gland health, this lovely young woman returned home excited and empowered that, with healthy changes, she could influence her sex life and marriage.

Let me also remind you men (Ladies, you already know this!) that female lubrication is enhanced by light touch and stimulation. Husbands, if you're constantly pursuing *On-In-and-Out sex*, don't be surprised if your wife regularly experiences vaginal dryness. It might benefit you to remember this simple rule: *If your wife's vagina isn't lubricated, she isn't ready!* Your sexual encounters will be greatly enhanced by an honest discussion of the amount of foreplay you are giving and the amount your wife needs to become lubricated. This foreplay might include light caressing, kissing and stroking which eventually lead to light clitoral and vaginal simulation. I think it's safe to say that women do not want to be "rubbed all over — in one spot." Pay attention to *all* of your wife's body and you'll be amazed by how she responds with lubrication!

PAINFUL PENETRATION DUE TO CONSTIPATION

Constipation is a problem for many people but most never consider how much it affects them sexually. It can be incredibly uncomfortable when a woman has hard or packed stool in her lower colon that is competing for room with her husband's penis. If this is an issue in your marriage, you need to have conversation with your spouse about timing and bowel function.

I often see new patients who are only moving their bowels every four to seven days, and it's no wonder they're uncomfortable! The first method of treatment is increasing water intake. Your water should come from a pure source, free of chemicals and additives. Eliminate or at least limit soft drinks, tea and coffee. Start your day with a warm or hot cup of water and a wedge of lemon. Squeeze the lemon into the water, let it soak, then drink the water and eat the lemon (not the peel). This morning procedure helps promote elimination and increases liver function at the same time. You should also increase fiber intake by eating a mixed green salad each day for lunch, sprinkled with sesame and sunflower seeds.[6] You may also use Celtic Sea Salt® on your greens, which is a great source of minerals. Let food be your medicine and don't become dependent on a colon evacuator.

Another common source of constipation is low thyroid function. If the natural remedies discussed above aren't helping considerably, you should have your thyroid tested (see Turn Up the Heat Chapter). Occasionally constipation results from liver stagnation, which would be accompanied by symptoms including bloating, varicose veins and even spider veins. In my experience,

---

6   If you have a problem with diverticulosis you may want to soak the seeds in water first to make them less irritating to your colon.

vein issues usually coincide with constipation as the liver grows congested due to decreased bowel movements.

I've also seen colon function normalize with the correction of spinal misalignment of the upper lumbar or lower back area. The nerves which exit the spinal cord in that region are partially responsible for transmitting communication from the brain to the colon and intestines. When that nerve flow is freed by a spinal adjustment, signals between the brain and colon are released to promote normal and comfortable excretory function.

LACK OF DESIRE FOR INTIMACY

I've observed almost epidemic proportions of low libido in nearly every adult sexually active age group. People who are exhausted are simply not interested in sexual intimacy. Your body will direct nutrients where they are most needed, and because you can survive without sex, your body gives it very low priority when other systems are suffering from exhaustion.

I generally discover that lack of desire is due to stress on the endocrine or hormone system. My first method of treatment is simple: Rest! I also have my patients take appropriate supplementation specific for their deficiencies and avoid sugar, refined carbohydrates, pastries, soda and processed foods.

POOR SELF IMAGE

The last sexual challenge that many women struggle with is a poor self image. Our society inundates women with magazines, television and movies that create an obsession with body perfection. The standards are completely unrealistic, but even that knowledge often isn't enough to stop women from comparing themselves to airbrushed images or anorexic models. The current obesity epidemic makes this unrealistic ideal even more of an impossibility for most women. It's no wonder then that discouraged women feel incredibly self conscious making love with the lights on when they are obsessing over every extra pound, stretch mark and grey hair.

Women may have legitimate reasons for concern if they are grossly obese or extremely unhealthy. The good news is there are many ways to make healthy changes that will benefit your health *and* your sex life! But ladies, I'd like to give you some secret insight into the inner workings of your husband's mind. When you head to the bedroom for lovemaking and take off your clothes, your husband is too focused and excited to be distracted by whatever physical flaws you may have. If feeling self conscious has been putting a damper on your sex life, it's time to sit down for a gentle and honest discussion about what you can do to make changes.

The most obvious change is the level of lighting in your bedroom. Your husband is probably very turned on by visual stimuli (You!), but maybe you can consider adjusting the lighting finding a happy medium that lets him enjoy your nakedness while at the same time allowing you more discretion. Another simple solution is to buy some lingerie that reveals your physical assets while covering areas you don't feel that confident about. With loving communication, couples can bring peace and security into their lovemaking.

CONCLUSION

There are many reasons you may not be able or desire to have sexual intimacy. Focus on one or two and make a plan to start treating them. Many solutions are simple and you'll be amazed by how quickly they promote good health and great sex!

JUST TELL ME WHAT TO DO

❑ Ladies, choose one area that has been problematic in your marriage. Start making small changes to bring improvement.

❑ Set aside a date night to discuss this challenge as a couple. Wives, have you communicated clearly to your spouse so they understand that you're not making excuses for resisting sexual advances? Husbands, have you been compassionate toward your wife as she deals with physical challenges?

❑ I recommend that every husband write these words on an index card and repeat them to your wife whenever you sense she doubts herself: "I love you for *who you are.*" No amount of their gray hair, stretch marks or length of years will change that. Ask God to help you love your wife unconditionally.

11

How It Works...
And When It Doesn't

Managing Erectile Dysfunction

Just like every other system in the body, the male sex organs are an engineering masterpiece. Glands, hormones, muscle, tissue and blood are all designed to work in tandem and create one of the most amazing and wonderful sensations available to men. There is no greater feeling than the awesome rush of an ejaculation as you look into the eyes of your wife.

I wish every couple could experience this wonderfully intimate moment each time they desired sexual intimacy; unfortunately, many men (and many wives!) are frustrated when male sex organs don't function as God intended. The cause may be neglect or ignorance but the result is the same: couples who are missing out on the exciting sexual relationship God wants them to experience.

This chapter will cover the following male sexual dysfunctions I commonly see and treat in my practice:

➢ erectile dysfunction

➢ ejaculation dysfunction

➢ diabetes-related dysfunction

➢ pain syndromes

> Peyronie's disease

> condom use and unfulfilled intercourse

Most men feel uncomfortable discussing their sexual desires and dysfunction issues with their wives; in fact, I often speak with women about their husband's challenges long before I actually have a frank conversation with the husband at all. I recently ran across an article in the Wall Street Journal Health Matters section entitled, "IS YOUR WIFE PUSHING YOU TO SEE A DOCTOR? READ THIS — AND GO." The article continued, "Doctors say wives are in a unique position to persuade their husbands to seek medical care. Erectile function is an important barometer of a man's health." I've discovered that women are usually more open, partly because they start talking about menstruation and sexuality in a clinical way early in their teens as puberty approaches. The conversation continues with their friends and spouse as they experience hormonal changes throughout their lifetime. In contrast, men's early sexual communication is likely to be locker room stories and boasting, which may or may not be factual. Men generally don't sit around discussing their challenges or inability to have sex, but these dysfunctions are deeply hurtful to a man's ego and sense of manhood. The inability to achieve a spontaneous erection during or before foreplay and penetration is like taking a weapon away from a soldier. A frank discussion of the problem — while absolutely necessary — takes trust, vulnerability, honesty, and humility by all parties involved.

When patients want to talk to me about sexual challenges they usually approach me the same way. With glassy eyes, they slowly lean forward and whisper, "Dr. Bob, I am having problems getting an erection," or, "Dr. Bob, I can get an erection…but I can't ejaculate." Quite often women will tell me the same thing about their husbands. Some wives tell me that their husband wakes them up three or four times in the night going to the bathroom to urinate. Then there are men who don't desire sexual intimacy, who have pain that prevents them from performing, or who won't give a reason for their lack of interest to their hurt, confused spouse. The good news is there is hope! Let's look in turn at each of the dysfunctions listed above and find out why things go wrong and what can be done to solve them.

ERECTILE DYSFUNCTION

Erectile dysfunction is by far the most common sexual dilemma I treat in men. This includes the complete inability to achieve an erection and the inability to maintain an erection when one is present.[1] The clinical criterion to diagnose this dysfunction is when it occurs more than twenty five percent of the time when you are aroused. It's been suggested that between 20 and up to 30 percent of men over forty years of age suffer from erectile dysfunction. This is a staggering statistic and a symptom of the declining health of our population. It's also a relatively new term; you will not find "erectile dysfunction" in older medical text books. The word "impotence" was used for this condition until the pharmaceutical industry created a drug to treat erection challenges. "Impotence" had negative connotations and drug companies wanted to de-stigmatize the condition so they made it more appealing by coining the term "Erectile Dysfunction" or "ED."

Erection challenges are a sign of the times and have become epidemic in our culture. As a result of poor diets filled with excessive processed convenience foods, lack of exercise and the increased used of stimulants, men have basically worn their bodies out. Increasingly, men are also exposed to estrogens in the water supply from the urine of patients consuming hormone replacement therapy or discarded medications dumped in the

---

1   Erectile dysfunction has nothing to do with the potency or presence of
    sperm. A man may be completely fertile though unable to arrive at an
    erection or maintain an adequate erection for penetration.

toilet. When a patient finally reluctantly brings up the subject with a medical doctor, it's far easier for that doctor to write a prescription and treat the symptom than coach the patient in lifestyle modification that will treat the *cause* of ED. This is a modern western cultural dilemma. Below is a list of common current conventional medical reasons for erectile dysfunction:

➢ Diseases and conditions such as diabetes, high blood pressure, heart or thyroid conditions, poor circulation, low testosterone, depression, and nerve damage from surgery.

➢ Medications such as blood pressure medications (beta-blockers), heart medication (such as digoxin), some peptic ulcer medications, sleeping pills and antidepressants.

➢ Nicotine, alcohol, and cocaine.[2]

➢ Stress, fear, anxiety and anger.

➢ Unrealistic sexual expectations which make intimacy a chore or task rather than a pleasure.

➢ Poor communication with your spouse.

➢ A "vicious cycle" of doubt, failure, or negative communications that reinforce the erection problem.

COMMON DIETARY AND STRUCTURAL FACTORS PRECIPITATING ERECTILE DYSFUNCTION

➢ Diets high in wheat and soy products depleting zinc. Zinc is necessary for many enzyme reactions to occur in the body, including prostate health, memory, blood sugar stress (zinc helps make insulin for blood sugar handling) and tissue healing.

---

2   Alcohol initially provokes desire but then inhibits the ability to physically follow through.

> Vegetarian diets high in copper are often low in zinc and contain inadequate complete proteins.

> Diets high in soy tend to add more estrogen factors antagonizing testosterone.

> Exposure to estrogen compounds in conventional meat and other products.

> Exposure to synthetic compounds that create a gallbladder/liver burden, including medications and industrial compounds.[3]

THE PHYSIOLOGY OF ERECTILE DYSFUNCTION

So just how does the erection mechanism work? The autonomic nervous system is the major component responsible for erections. This system functions just like it sounds: automatically. What a brilliant design; we don't have to think about breathing, swallowing, having bowel movements and a whole host of other normal body functions that are necessary for life. This automatic system is divided into two major parts that work in unison with each other: the sympathetic and the parasympathetic nervous systems. Simply stated, the sympathetic system speeds you up, and the parasympa- thetic slows you down. Ideally, they are balanced to allow your body to work flawlessly. You can think of these nervous systems as the gas and the brake on a car; at times you need to accelerate and at other times you need to brake.

> Unfortunately, in most of the sexually compromised patients I treat, the sympathetic is on overdrive and dominates the parasympathetic nervous system. The reason this dominance is so destructive sexually is because the parasympathetic system is responsible for achieving and maintaining erections.

---

3   You can get a list of environmental toxins from the American Cancer Society's webpage.

Unfortunately, in most of the sexually compromised patients I treat, the sympathetic is on overdrive and dominates the parasympathetic nervous system. The reason this dominance is so destructive sexually is because the parasympathetic system is responsible for achieving and maintaining erections. Lowered parasympathetic activity leads to lowered erection function. Lowered erection function leads to diminished sexual activity. Diminished sexual activity leads to unhappy, frustrated, disconnected husbands and wives. You get the picture.

The sympathetic nervous system's dominance is commonly due to poor diet choices with too much sugar and artificial stimulants, lack of exercise, high levels of stress and no time to rest.

ERECTILE DYSFUNCTION DUE TO MISALIGNMENT

The parasympathetic nervous system has a direct connection from the brain to the penis by way of the Vagus nerve. When the nerve is compressed, signals to achieve and/or maintain an erection are partially or fully blocked. These compressions, or subluxations, may occur in the neck where the nerve first exits the brain or in the lumbar or sacral area of the lower back where the message is delivered to the genitals. Daily events can precipitate subluxation: poor posture, poor sleep habits, motor vehicle accidents, stressful work conditions, exercise and sport injuries, and gravity. With regular spinal adjustments, many of my patients suffering from ED have reported naturally-occurring, consistent erections — without the use of medication.

Stimulation of the Vagus nerve has also been used by conventional medical practitioners to decrease depression, creating an interesting correlation between erectile dysfunction and depression. While researching medical information for erection challenges, I discovered that some institutions are implanting Vagus nerve stimulators to treat both depression and erectile issues. This strongly suggests an association between the nervous system, depression and erectile dysfunction.

If you are suffering with erection issues you should always have your lower pelvis and spine assessed and corrected accordingly before you consider taking any medication with serious side effects. I've had many smiling wives of my ED patients come to the office thanking us for improving their sex life while avoiding the negative side effects common from most erectile dysfunction drugs.

MEDICATION SIDE EFFECTS AND ERECTILE DYSFUNCTION

Erectile dysfunction is a side effect of many common drugs. Three significant and highly-prescribed drugs are beta-blockers, antidepressants, and statins. We'll discuss each in detail.

Beta Blockers

Beta blockers are used to treat high blood pressure, migraine headaches, anxiety, heart palpitations and glaucoma. These drugs interfere with the flow of blood to the penis by blocking the action of the chemical transmitters that communicate between nerves and other tissues.

High blood pressure is very common in the Western world, caused largely by poor diets and stress. Weight is not always an accurate measure for who likely suffers from high blood pressure; I have seen very heavy individuals with normal pressure and thin folks with high blood pressure.

Today's pharmaceutical community continues to lower the numbers which are considered normal for blood pressure; I sense they are doing this to sell more medication. Before you treat with medication, try some natural methods to lower your blood pressure. First make sure your diet is providing ample calcium. Do you get cold sores, leg cramps at night and colds easily? These are all signs of inadequate calcium. I encourage my patients to take calcium in the form of calcium citrate or lactate. Calcium helps relax the very tight blood vessels that may increase your blood pressure. You could also incorporate kelp and black cohash, two herbs with a history of naturally lowering blood pressure.

Eliminating refined grain sweetened carbohydrates (pastries, donuts, muffins etc.) from the diet is another natural treatment, because carbohydrates increase insulin, which causes sodium to be retained in the system and elevates blood pressure. Mung beans (commonly used to make bean sprouts) soaked in hot water and consumed daily are also a helpful natural remedy.[4]

You can drink two 1-ounce servings of organic pomegranate juice a day. Additionally, increased water intake from a pure source results in thinning of the blood and lowered pressure. My patients have also experienced erectile improvement by using Celtic Sea Salt® and alfalfa.

Antidepressants

Many of the new patients coming into the office suffering from erectile dysfunction are taking prescription medications for depression. The risk and severity of sexual side effects depends on the individual and the specific type and dose of antidepressant, but common sexual side effects include reduced sexual desire, erectile dysfunction and difficulty achieving orgasm or ejaculation. Following is a list of antidepressants that may be in your medicine cabinet, causing your erection difficulties:

---

4   Soak one tablespoon of mung beans in hot water and drink the water. Add eight ounces of water back in the beans and repeat twice during the day. At the third session, drink the water and also eat the beans. Source: *The Scientific Validation of Herbal Medicine* by Daniel Mowery.

> Bupropion (Wellbutrin), a norepinephrine and dopamine reuptake inhibitor (NDRI) Nefazodone,

> A combined reuptake inhibitor and receptor blocker Mirtazapine (Remeron),

> A tetracyclic antidepressant Duloxetine (Cymbalta),

> A serotonin and norepinephrine reuptake inhibitor Selective serotonin reuptake inhibitors (SSRIs) — such as fluoxetine (Prozac), paroxetine (Paxil) and sertraline (Zoloft) — all have a high rate of sexual side effects. Some research suggests that Paxil is more likely to cause sexual dysfunction than are other SSRIs.

> Tricyclic antidepressants — such as amitriptyline, clomipramine (Anafranil), amoxapine and desipramine (Norpramin) — have a lower rate of sexual dysfunction than do SSRIs.

Exactly how these antidepressants interfere with sexual desire and function remains the subject of ongoing debate and investigation. Unproven theories abound; for example, some blame the sedating effect of certain antidepressants for dampening sexual desire. Others speculate these antidepressants cause chemical changes in the parts of the brain regulating sexual desire and function. Complicating all of this is the effect of depression itself in decreasing sexual desire and function.

It's impossible to predict which individuals are most likely to develop sexual side effects while taking an antidepressant. In some cases, sexual side effects may improve once your body adjusts to the medication; but in other patients, sexual side effects may last for the duration of treatment. If you experience sexual side effects while taking an antidepressant, consider these strategies.

Talk to your conventional doctor about the possibility of changing your dose of anti-depressant medication. You may want to consider taking a medication requiring only a once-a-day dose, and schedule sexual activity before taking that dose if you are not in a position to discontinue antidepressant medications at this time. You should also contact an experienced natural healthcare provider for assistance with your diet. Consider having a thyroid test to determine whether there are other natural ways to treat your depression.

How well these strategies work depends on the specific drug and your individual circumstances. If sexual side effects are troublesome, talk to your doctor before discontinuing your medication. Conventional medical physicians are traditionally of the mindset that any approach other than the pharmaceutical protocol is unsafe. My experience indicates that if you are motivated to change your diet, exercise, and take the supplements your body needs, you will be pleasantly surprised. You can be depression *and* antidepressant free!

Depression can be precipitated by many factors including insufficient amounts of Omega-3 oils found in foods such as flax oil, walnuts and greens. Consuming an abundance of snack or convenience foods with trans-fat or partially hydrogenated oils is also problematic; trans fats interfere with the production of DHA, a long-chain fat needed for optimal brain health and commonly deficient in depressed patients.

I have witnessed depressed patients improve when their thyroid is assessed and supplemented with iodine and tyrosine. Tyrosine is an amino acid or protein building-block.

I have successfully treated depressed patients by including marine and animal proteins in their diet, especially turkey and tuna. I also encourage chicken thighs and legs (with healthy fat which is beneficial for the brain) and adding whole food B vitamins.

Of course, there are causes of depression which are purely psychological such as poor self image, stress, abuse, anger and un-forgiveness. If you suspect your depression may have a psychological as well as physiological component, seek out a qualified Christian counselor.

Statin Drugs

Statin drugs are marketed as a treatment for everything from lowering cholesterol to preventing cancer. These drugs have very chilling side effects that include erectile dysfunction and liver disease. They may also cause increased body pain and create a deficiency of Coenzyme Q10. Statin drugs work by sabotaging cholesterol metabolism in the body. Cholesterol has a bad reputation because its role in human physiology is not understood. In reality, cholesterol is neither good nor bad; it's a vital component in many important functions in the body including the production of steroid hormones.[5] Without cholesterol your cell membranes won't function like they should and your adrenal glands will be unable to produce testosterone, progesterone, estrogen and cortisone. High cholesterol levels only become problematic when they are elevated; this is usually a result of cholesterol's normal response to inflammation in the body due to poor eating habits. Avoiding partially hydrogenated or trans fats and lowering sugar intake is helpful in controlling cholesterol levels. Tragically, the public has bought into low fat/no fat diet fads which are loaded with deadly man-made trans fats. For years the medical community promoted these harmful diets and people were simply ignorant of the proper role of cholesterol in good health.[6] Eating an apple each day can lower

---

5   Elevated cholesterol levels are not the primary cause of heart attacks; many people who suffer a heart attack have normal cholesterol levels. Inflammation of the vessel wall is the primary cause of heart failure.

6   I discuss the role of cholesterol in great detail in *Dr. Bob's Trans-Fat Survival Guide: Why No-Fat, Low-Fat, Trans-Fat is KILLING You.*

your cholesterol thirteen percent, and you can lower cholesterol forty percent by adding beets to your diet.

TREATING ERECTILE DYSFUNCTION

After an assessment of ED is made, the first method of treatment should be spinal corrective care. Many patients respond quickly to spinal manipulation that restores proper nervous system function to their genitals.

Adrenal fatigue is the next culprit, which is treated by cutting sugar out of a patient's diet. (As you will read in the Adrenal Gland Chapter, over-consumption of sugar stresses the adrenal glands' ability to make sex hormones and transmitters.) To stop the sugar craving, supplement with whole food chromium, a mineral commonly deficient in those who crave sweets and an herb called gymnema which takes away the taste for sweets. Cutting out sugar is absolutely essential if you want to give your adrenal glands any possible chance of being restored. This includes sweet fruits such as bananas, raisins, grapes, pineapple and any dried fruit. (Pears, plums and apples are an awesome fruit choice any day of the week.) You should also avoid energy drinks loaded with stimulants which stress adrenal function.

Zinc deficiencies are quite common in men with ED, causing enlargement of the prostrate and frequent urination. Zinc plays a role in memory, the production of insulin, healing, the immune system and about ninety other functions. White spots on the fingernails are a common symptom of low zinc levels, as are large facial pores. In my office we incorporate a zinc taste test and supplement with a liquid product accordingly, eventually changing to a dry tablet.[7] Wheat and soy should be avoided as they tend to deplete the body of necessary zinc.

---

7   Read more about the zinc taste test at www.druglessdoctor.com.

Iodine and Tyrosine supplements are used when thyroid function is the cause of ED. There are also herbs available for treatment. The herb Tribulus helps stimulate the body's ability to create testosterone, increasing libido. My patients also routinely take a whole food product or herbal supplement for hormonal balance and increased function, available at www.druglessdoc tor.com.

Finally, appropriate lifestyle modifications should be made. Herbs and supplements are beneficial, but the ultimate goal is to help the body function fully with whole foods and the elimination of toxic habits.

NOCTURNAL ERECTIONS

Before we move on to ejaculation dysfunction, let me mention something here about nocturnal erections. It's possible for a man to have three to five erections during the night, each one lasting up to thirty minutes. (You may want to take advantage of the moment!) If you wake up in the middle of the night or in the morning with an erection, it means your body is functioning correctly. It may also be a sign that your daytime erectile dysfunction has psychological roots rather than physiological ones. The problem may be stress related, due to performance anxiety, or the result of marital difficulties stemming from other issues. You may also experience difficulty getting an erection if you have recently ejaculated or have had multiple sexual encounters over a short period of time. You may desire to have sex, but your body has a refractory period during which it replenishes sperm and seminal fluid and the ability to achieve an erection is diminished. This is a normal part of the sexual cycle.

EJACULATION DYSFUNCTION

As we've discussed, the nervous systems that work in tandem are the parasympathetic (slows you down) and sympathetic (speeds you up). The parasympathetic system is in charge of achieving and maintaining erections, while the sympathetic nervous system is in charge of ejaculation. Because these functions are controlled by separate systems, it's completely possible to have one without the other. (A normal erection and the inability to ejaculate, or the ability to ejaculate with a very soft erection.) Optimally, the two systems are well balanced so that both erection and ejaculation can be achieved at the appropriate time. The adrenal glands release chemical transmitters which stimulate the sympathetic nervous system for ejaculation. These significant transmitters are generally low or depleted in individuals who experience ejaculation dysfunction.

To manage these challenges naturally you should eliminate sugar from your diet, avoid processed foods, minimize stress and eat whole foods. Alcohol intake should be moderate and if you smoke, you should start a plan to quit immediately.

Another ejaculation dysfunction I commonly see is a result of nerve compression. The sensations of an orgasm travel to the brain along a nerve that exits the spine in the lumbar area of the back. Fully experienced, the nerve impulses create an electrifying sensation throughout a man's body, including an endorphin rush and a momentary high. The signals quickly travel from the penis to the brain and back, transmitting pleasure and the cues that lead to ejaculation. I wish I could more fully explain to women just how wonderful this sensation is. It's the reason that physically and emotionally healthy men desire passionately to recreate this feeling on a regular basis with their wives! (Some men may even experience "goose bumps" as they ejaculate — the sympathetic nervous system's response to excitation.) But because this area is often misaligned or injured, the compression of the nerve inhibits the orgasm nerve impulses resulting in less powerful orgasms and ejaculations. This is reason enough for every husband to see a chiropractor trained in spinal manipulation!

DIABETES AND SEXUAL DYSFUNCTION

Diabetes is the third-highest killer of people in our country; I can even foresee it becoming number one as a result of our society's addiction to sugar, lack of exercise and obesity. The complications of diabetes can affect every tissue in the body. Patients who present a history of diabetes or even pre-diabetic tendencies are more apt to be pain-sensitive, have higher rates of infection and generally seem to suffer from a large variety of health issues. Diabetes interferes with the movement and use of fuel (glucose) in the body, gradually decreasing pancreatic function. This increases insulin levels, which in turn creates inflammation in the body and reduced blood flow. Erections are built and maintained with blood flow in the genitals, so you can see how this disease plays a large role in erectile health.

Natural treatments for diabetes-related erectile dysfunction would include minimizing refined grain products with sugar. I always encourage my patients to exercise with weights, resistive bands, training equipment and aerobic activity. Losing weight is a step in the right direction because weight loss is critical for long-term blood sugar control.

PAIN SYNDROMES

I treat a variety of pain syndromes in my practice. Back and pelvic pain prevent many couples from having intercourse. Even if they are capable of intercourse, pain often limits the variety of sexual positions they can enjoy. Varying sexual positions keeps intimacy fresh and exciting, and a couple's relationship is bound to suffer when they don't have this wonderful variety available.

If you experience spinal pain during intercourse, schedule an assessment by a skilled chiropractor and also seek an experienced trainer to assist you in toning and strengthening your core muscles. Deb and I have worked out for years, and I'm absolutely certain that the strength we've gained as a result has enhanced our ability to engage in and enjoy intimate sexual contact.

I've had many patients come to my office complaining of pain radiating into the groin from their back. Three of these men were actually scheduled to have their left testicle medically removed as a solution to the problem; quite a drastic solution if you ask me! All three men had misaligned pelvic bones. With appropriate assessment and spinal correction, their testicle pain went away. Each returned to their physician and was relieved to have avoided the surgery. If you are suffering from this pain syndrome, your pelvic alignment should be assessed by a health care provider who is skilled in natural spinal manipulation. Always rule out pathology, but seek a natural treatment first and foremost.

Pain may also be a culprit in places other than the reproductive organs. I recently had a consultation with a husband and wife. The husband was quite distraught because every time his wife had an orgasm she would develop a severe migraine. You can imagine that this was interfering with their sexual relationship! She completed a very detailed symptom survey form and I determined her pituitary gland was not up to full function. We supported the gland with a natural product and her migraines went away.

PEYRONIE'S DISEASE (Also referred to as Bent Penis)

Another sexual challenge becoming more prevalent is Peyronie's disease. This condition results in painful, hardened, cord-like lesions (scar tissue known as "plaques") and abnormal curvature of the penis when erect. In addition, narrowing and/or shortening of the penis may occur. Pain felt in the early stages of the disease often resolves in twelve to eighteen months. Erectile dysfunction, in varying degrees, often accompanies these symptoms in its later stages. The condition may make painful and/or difficult, though many men report satisfactory intercourse in spite of the disease. Although it can affect men of any race and age, it's most commonly seen in Caucasian males above the age of 40. Peyronie's is not contagious, nor is it related in any way to cancer. The disease only affects men and is confined to the penis.

About thirty percent of men with Peyronie's disease develop fibrosis in other elastic tissues of the body, such as on the hand or foot, including Dupuytren's contracture of the hand (is a contracture of the hand where the bend towards the palm and cannot be straightened). An increased incidence in genetically related males suggests a genetic component. From my experience I've noticed two common causes: high copper found on mineral tissue hair analysis resulting in adhesions, and low iodine found on the iodine loading test with lower than midline values seen on the T3 and T4 thyroid panel test. (See the Turning up the Heat Chapter for more insight on facilitating normal tissue function.) If you're experiencing any of the symptoms of Peyronie's you should see an experienced health care provider.

I would suggest having a mineral tissue hair analysis to determine copper and zinc ratios. High copper levels increase the risk of tissue binding adhesions as discussed above. Heightened zinc intake can bring copper to a more normal state. You should also avoid wheat, soy and sugar.

CONDOM USE AND UNFULFILLED INTERCOURSE

This form of male sexual challenge is rarely discussed but has an extremely large impact on the sexual psyche of a man and the sexual health of a couple. When God designed the act of intercourse, his intentions were for an incredibly intimate flesh-to-flesh encounter; that two "...shall become one flesh."[8]

---

8   Genesis 2:24

One form of birth control inhibits this flesh-to-flesh encounter: the condom.

Let me share my own experience with you. Deb used birth control pills the first six years of our marriage. Looking back, I'm sure the pill altered her body chemistry, including her hormone balance, but we really didn't know any better back then and to be honest, our sex life was great in every other regard.[9] We decided to start a family and stopped using oral contraceptives. After our first son was born, Deb and I agreed that she would not go back on the birth control pill. For the next four years between her pregnancies we used condoms for contraception. Deb didn't mind this method, mainly because we threw the condom away and she didn't have to deal with my semen flowing out of her for the next couple of hours. My experience, however, was completely different.

Condom use over those four years had a drastic impact on our marriage, though it wasn't until years later that I was able to look back and recognize all that was occurring. After years of skin-to-skin intercourse with my wife, putting on a condom and losing that intimate contact took the spark out of our sex life for me. We were still having intercourse, but it was like the intimacy of the act was gone. You see, God knew what he was doing when he created the male and female sexual organs. Men have an internal explosion of emotional sexual feelings with intimate skin-to-skin intercourse. I've attempted to explain this to Deb but it's almost like I don't have the words for it. A physical and arousing bonding called "sexual transmutation" occurs during this most intimate act that becomes even more intense as a man makes passionate love to a woman and then ejaculates inside of

---

9   Refer to the Hormone Chapter for more information on the pill's hormonal effects.

her. Intercourse becomes much more than contact between sexual organs; the meeting of flesh actually fuses a couple together — mind, body and spirit. This is what God is speaking of when he talks about two becoming one flesh. A condom insulates partners from each other and from the skin-to-skin contact that they desire and God intended.

This constant lack of skin-to-skin intimacy with Deb had enormous repercussions. I suddenly felt disconnected from her sexually. Even though we continued to have sex, I felt like we weren't really being intimate. It drove me crazy, and it also drove me to drink! I drowned my pity party with alcohol, which only compounded our marital problems because I was nearly always high on "spirits" and not the Holy Spirit. Of course, having sex with a drunk wasn't very appealing to Deb and soon she felt as sexually distant as I did.

I'm not saying that condoms were the reason I drank, but I *was* very frustrated. We had very limited sexual time together and drifted far apart. The alcohol temporarily distracted me from those frustrations but also decreased our sexual and emotional involvement. Deb was not pleased with me or the choices I was making, but she hung in there by the grace of God. I accepted the Lord into my life the year after our youngest son was born, and it took four more years but I was finally supernaturally released from alcohol addiction by the power of the Holy Spirit. I know if I had continued my excessive alcohol consumption we more than likely would have divorced.

After our second son was born I had a vasectomy. It was one of the wisest decisions we have ever made! It enables us to have very spontaneous sex without hesitation, and we don't have to stop and search for a condom or take the time to put one on. If you're currently using condoms, have a frank and honest discussion about the impact they are having on your sexual relationship. If either partner is suffering from a lack of skin-to-skin contact, discuss another method of birth control.

You may be struggling with one or more of the conditions addressed in this chapter, but be encouraged. You *can* have the mutually fulfilling sex life that God intends and you desire! Start by choosing one or two ways to naturally treat whatever is holding you back and ask the Lord to bless your efforts. He is willing and able to bless your health, your sexual function, and your marriage!

JUST TELL ME WHAT TO DO

Journal what you eat and drink for one week. Do you recognize a pattern of sweets, grains and soda? If you do, schedule a family meeting and agree together to slowly incorporate healthy choices of organic vegetables and protein into your diet. Your well-being as well as your family's health will improve!

- ❑ Drink water from a pure source.
- ❑ Are you depressed, have high blood pressure or a history of heart disease? Find a proactive natural health care provider who can coach you from a prescription-based mind-set to one that is a natural health and wellness way of life.
- ❑ Walk a minimum of twenty minutes daily with your spouse or find another form of exercise that you can do together.
- ❑ If you drink alcohol and have erectile challenges, consider cutting back or quitting altogether.
- ❑ Review the Adrenal and Thyroid Chapters.
- ❑ Take advantage of nocturnal erections if you have ED difficulties during the day.
- ❑ Search for a contraceptive method that facilitates skin-to-skin contact.

While we're talking about skin-to-skin contact, here's something for you to ponder: When a man ejaculates inside his wife his seminal fluid is absorbed by her vaginal cells. Because it contains highs levels of protein, semen is a source of cellular nutrition and a woman's body will absorb the protein in her husband's ejaculate. In natural health care, using the proteins (the RNA and DNA) of one animal to treat another is called cell therapy or glandular therapy. After prolonged ejaculations (I'm talking about a number of years), a woman may actually start to take on some physical characteristics of her spouse. Look at the couples you know who have been married for a long time and you may notice they're beginning to resemble each other!

12

Your Reserve Tank for Sexual Function

The conventional medical model is very compartmentalized, breaking the human body down into single systems. While this concept is useful for instructional purposes, in reality, our systems don't function independently of each other. Your body is a complex, *interdependent* network of systems whose functions impact each other in profound ways. Unfortunately, western medicine has generally treated sexual dysfunction with medication and ignored the delicate balance of all of the components involved in sexual health. One key player in that system is the adrenal glands, which often play a role in erectile dysfunction, vaginal dryness and suppressed libido.

I want to encourage you to read this chapter slowly in order to fully grasp all the truths it contains. Each new piece of information adds to the foundation of personal health and optimal sexual function.

Located on top of the kidneys, the adrenal glands are about the size of walnuts. As an important member of the endocrine system, the glands work closely with the pituitary, pancreas and thyroid. One of their many functions is to help the body cope with stress. For our purposes, we'll focus on the role these potent glands play in sexual health and function.

The adrenal glands are comprised of a large outer portion called the cortex and the smaller inner portion, the medulla. The cortex and medulla have different but very significant roles in sexual function. The medulla secretes epinephrine and norepinephrine, two hormones responsible for the body's fight or flight response to stress. The cortex produces over 50 different types of hormones in three major classes:

> Gluccorticoids

> Mineralcorticoids

> Androgens

The most important glucocorticoid is cortisol. When cortisol production is too low, the body's ability to deal with stress is markedly reduced. We will discuss the important role of cortisol in further detail later in this chapter. Mineralcorticoids such as aldosterone (which is a hormone that causes the tubules of the kidneys to retain sodium and water) modulate the delicate balance of minerals in the cells, especially sodium and potassium, and play a part in blood pressure regulation. Stress increases the release of aldosterone, causing sodium retention. The result is water retention and high blood pressure. (When high blood pressure is treated with prescription medication, which is the norm in our society, a common side effect is erectile dysfunction.) The stress-induced release of aldosterone also results in a loss of potassium and magnesium, which wreaks havoc on your body. Magnesium is involved in many enzymatic reactions throughout multiple systems; low magnesium plays a role in a variety of serious conditions including cardiac arrhythmias, uterine fibroids, osteoporosis and constipation.

The adrenal cortex produces sex hormones in small but **potent** amounts. (See Figure One.) An exception is DHEA, a weak androgenic hormone. DHEA, together with testosterone and estrogen, are made from pregnenolone, which in turn comes from cholesterol.

Pregnenolone also leads to the production of progesterone and is one of the transition steps in the production of cortisol. Pregnenolone is therefore one of the significant intermediate hormones being produced in the hormonal cascade. Prolonged deficiencies in pregnenolone will lead to reduction of both glucocorticoids (cortisol) and mineralcorticoids (aldosterone).

Adrenal Glands

Steroid Hormone Synthesis Pathways

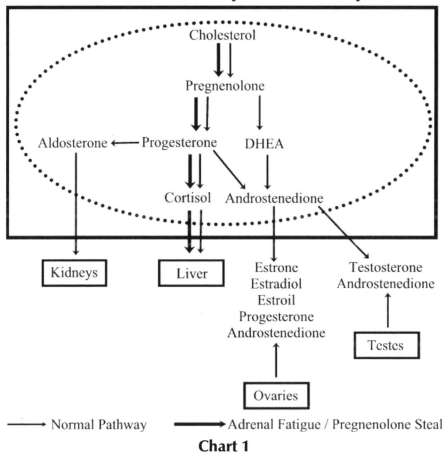

Chart 1

Cortisol is a very significant hormone, protecting the body from excessive daily pressure by:

Normalizing Blood Sugar — Cortisol increases blood sugar levels in the body, providing the energy necessary for the fight or flight response to danger. Cortisol works in tandem with insulin from the pancreas to provide adequate glucose to the cells for energy. More stress requires more energy, which explains why you crave refined carbohydrates and sweets when you are stressed. In adrenal fatigue, more cortisol is secreted during the early stages of stress until eventually the adrenal glands become exhausted and cortisol output is reduced. Blood sugar balance is disrupted, cholesterol is likely to increase, and you may experience more pain throughout your body. All of this occurs because your body is caught in the vicious and demanding cycle of producing pregnenelone, which in turn increases cortisol and keeps your body in a state of constant agitation.

Anti-inflammatory response — Cortisol — is a powerful anti-inflammatory agent. When you experience a minor injury or a muscle strain, your body's inflammatory cascade is initiated, leading to swelling and redness (commonly seen when an ankle is sprained or from an insect bite). Cortisol is secreted as a part of the anti-inflammatory response. Its objective is to remove and prevent swelling and redness of nearly all tissues. These anti-inflammatory responses prevent mosquito bites from enlarging, eyes from swelling due to allergies, etc.

Immune system suppression — People with high cortisol levels have suppressed immune systems. Cortisol influences cells that participate in the immune reaction, especially white blood cells. Cortisol suppresses white blood cells and other "fighter cells" whose purpose is to protect the body from threats such as bacteria, fungus, viruses and cancer. Lowered immunity results in increased sickness and disease.

Physiology of stress — People with adrenal fatigue cannot tolerate stress and are likely to succumb to severe nervous tension. As their stress increases, progressively higher levels of cortisol are required. When the cortisol level cannot rise in response to the situation at hand (job stress, hectic schedules, financial concerns, chronic marital or family challenges), it is impossible to maintain a body that is fully prepared to react appropriately to stress.

Cortisol sustains life through opposite but related regulatory actions: releasing and activating the body's defense mechanisms and shutting down and modifying those same mechanisms to prevent damage or cell loss.

The adrenal glands are directed via the hypothalamus-pituitary-adrenal, the HPA loop or axis as discussed in the Hormone Chapter. There is an existing negative feedback loop which governs the amount of adrenal hormones secreted under normal circumstances. For example, the HPA axis adjusts cortisol levels according to the body's need via a hormone called Adrenal Corticotrophic Hormone (ACTH) which is secreted from the pituitary gland in response to signals from the hypothalamus, your body's CEO.

When the ACTH attaches to the walls of the adrenal glands, a chain reaction occurs within the cell. This leads to the release of cholesterol, which is manufactured into pregnenolone, the first hormone in the adrenal metabolism (See Chart 1). Subsequently, cortisol is released into the blood stream and moves throughout the body and back to the hypothalamus where it is measured. This completes the negative feedback loop. In the human hormonal system, the negative feedback loop is designed to limit the production of each hormone.

This whole process is an amazing part of your physiology and a testimony to God's awesome creative power. When cared for, your body is kept in a constant state of homeostasis, or balance. Unfortunately, many people exist in a constant state of prolonged *stress*, and the increased cortisol levels that result blunt the negative feedback response. The delicate balance between the sympathetic and parasympathetic nervous systems is threatened as the sympathetic revs up to address the impending danger that increased cortisol levels have announced. (The sympathetic and parasympathetic nervous systems are explained in detail at the end of this chapter.) As the parasympathetic system is pushed aside, so are many of its sexual functions, including vaginal lubrication and the ability to produce and maintain an erection.

A body that is constantly flooded with the stress hormone cortisol is a body in distress. Why the constant stress? There are multiple reasons. A diet full of sugary foods creates a challenge for the adrenal glands. A stressful job, family problems, a high-paced life — all of these lead to increased cholesterol, which, when called on, jumpstarts the production of that useful but lethal hormone, cortisol. Taking cholesterol-lowering medications often leads to erectile dysfunction. One problem is "solved" and a new one is created.[1]

Stress, then, induces the following responses in your body:

➤ Reduced insulin sensitivity, reduced glucose (or blood sugar) utilization and increased blood sugar lead to diabetes and the potential for erectile dysfunction if the disease is not properly managed.

➤ Reduced natural killer cells in the body lead to infections such as herpes, yeast overgrowth, bacteria and viral infections. Women may experience chronic vaginal yeast infestation and men may develop genital rash and fungus on the toes or athlete's foot.

---

1   It's important to understand that avoiding red meat, cheese and fat may help reduce cholesterol, but a sugary diet and the inability to handle stress will continue to keep cholesterol levels elevated.

➢ Increased loss in bone mass as calcium absorption is blocked and demineralization of bone occurs, results in osteoporosis.

➢ Increased fat accumulation around the waist and protein breakdown lead to loss of muscle tone and the inability to lose weight.

➢ Increased water and salt retention lead to high blood pressure.[2]

➢ Estrogen saturation and/or dominance. This condition can lead to uterine fibroids, premenstrual syndrome (PMS) and breast cancer. Estrogen creates an environment for tender breasts and heavy periods, which are likely to interfere with sexual intimacy. Estrogen saturation in men may result in prostate challenges.

Now you know what a hormonal reaction to stress looks like on paper, but what does it look like in real life? Imagine you're at work and your boss raises his voice to you. Here's what happens in your body from a hormonal perspective as the stress response kicks in:

➢ Your hypothalamus signals your pituitary gland to release Adrenal Corticotrophic Hormone (ACTH).

➢ The ACTH stimulates the adrenal medulla to secrete epinephrine and the adrenal cortex to secrete cortisol and other hormones.

➢ The epinephrine increases your heart rate.

➢ The cortisol causes increased sweat production.

➢ Both cortisol and epinephrine increase muscle tension.

➢ Digestion slows as blood is diverted away from organs that are less important to the fight or flight response.

---

2   As noted previously, the use of medication to treat high blood pressure can result in erectile dysfunction.

➤ The sympathetic nervous system is on high-alert, dominating the parasympathetic nervous system. In an agitated state, your body <u>is more concerned with survival</u> than ancillary functions like sexual encounters, which are less essential in a state of emergency.

You arrive home after a tough day, and just when sexual intimacy might be a wonderful release of tension, the last thing your body wants to do or is capable of doing is performing the sexual act!

WOMEN AND ADRENALS

The adrenal glands contribute about 35 percent of female hormones pre-menopausal and almost 50 percent post-menopausal. Without properly functioning adrenal glands, full term pregnancy cannot occur. From my experience, lowered progesterone increases the rate of miscarriage, especially in second pregnancies.

Women today often experience adrenal fatigue by the time they reach their mid-thirties or early forties due to stressful lifestyles; it is not unusual to see this in the early twenties. I have even treated women in their early twenties who suffer from vaginal dryness and painful intercourse in part because of altered adrenal function.

Post-menopausal women may also experience hair loss due to adrenal fatigue. Hair loss may be a sign of excessive androgen (male) hormone production.[3] I have also observed elevated testosterone levels in women who have cysts on their ovaries and liver congestion.

---

3   Hair loss can also be a result of low thyroid function and the lack of certain minerals.

Stress is primarily regulated by our adrenal glands. In early stages of adrenal fatigue, the body attempts to neutralize the stress by higher cortisol production. However, when too much cortisol is produced, it will have multiple adverse effects. For example, cortisol blocks progesterone receptors, making them less responsive to progesterone. Progesterone normally produced by the adrenals comes to a halt in favor of cortisol. Insufficient progesterone production leads to estrogen dominance. The results are premenstrual syndrome (PMS), fibroids, and the early onset of menopausal symptoms. Heavy menstrual bleeding may even cause relatively young women to undergo ablation (cauterizing the uterus lining) or hysterectomy.

> **Insufficient progesterone production leads to estrogen dominance. The results are premenstrual syndrome (PMS), fibroids, and the early onset of menopausal symptoms.**

Too quickly, women jump at hormonal supplementation to treat all of these maladies, but the truth is that optimal adrenal function is usually possible and should be the first step in treatment. In fact, hormone replacement alone often treats the symptoms without addressing the overall health of the adrenal glands. It becomes a band-aid that is often ineffective in the long run.

The adrenal normalization process begins with investigating and eliminating stressors. Stressors are often chronic in nature and can be related to lifestyle, diet and emotional health. Women with adrenal exhaustion should normalize their adrenal functions with adequate sleep, proper diet,[4] nutritional supplementation, detoxification, *Dr. Bob's Drugless Guide to Detoxification* and elimination of outside stressors *before* considering progesterone therapy.

---

4   See dietary suggestions in the Page Fundamental Diet Appendix 3.

If you want more insight into your hormonal health, I strongly suggest saliva testing of your estrogen, progesterone, testosterone, cortisol and DHEA levels. Men should also have saliva testing to determine their testosterone, DHEA and cortisol levels. This testing method is a simple and easy way to start your program of hormonal restoration.

1 Peter 5:7 says that we're able to cast all of our anxieties, worries and concerns on God because He cares for us affectionately and watches over us. The peace that comes from running to God with all of your problems is a wonderful first step in combating any kind of physical, mental or emotional fatigue. Because your body and spirit are connected, emotional calmness translates into a body that is more able to relax and respond to all the demands life puts on it. We strongly encourage you to maintain your spirit as mindfully as you maintain your body!

MEN AND ADRENAL HEALTH

Women have a larger network of hormones requiring harmony than men do, but men can just as easily experience adrenal fatigue. Men commonly work at high-stress jobs, consume diets lacking in good nutrition, and may live life more recklessly than their female counterparts. All of these challenge the hormonal system and the result is dominance by the sympathetic nervous system.

As men age and experience chronic stress, their bodies become less effective producing the necessary steroids for sexual function. If your belly is 40 inches or more and your legs and arms are starting to look like toothpicks, your androgens are not at a sufficient level to promote muscle strength and integrity. This is a very common and serious condition prevalent in our culture. Men over forty-five think they are nineteen and yet they have the hormonal capacity of a seventy-year-old. And we wonder why men need to take a pill to get an erection!

THE ADRENAL GLAND ASSESSMENT

Do you experience…

- ☐ Difficulty getting up in the morning
- ☐ Continuing fatigue which is not relieved by sleep and rest
- ☐ Lethargy, lack of energy to perform normal daily activities
- ☐ Sugar cravings
- ☐ Salt cravings
- ☐ Allergies
- ☐ Digestion problems
- ☐ Increased effort needed for everyday tasks
- ☐ Decreased interest in sex
- ☐ Decreased ability to handle stress
- ☐ Increased time needed to recover from illness, injury or traumas
- ☐ Light-headed or dizzy when standing up quickly
- ☐ Low mood
- ☐ Less enjoyment or happiness with life
- ☐ Increased PMS
- ☐ Symptoms worsen if meals are skipped or inadequate
- ☐ Thoughts are less focused, brain fog
- ☐ Poor memory
- ☐ Decreased tolerance for stress, noise, disorder
- ☐ Not really awake until after 10:00 a.m.
- ☐ Afternoon slump between 3:00 p.m. and 4:00 p.m.
- ☐ Feel better after supper
- ☐ Get a "second wind" in the evening and stay up late

- ☐ Decreased productivity
- ☐ Have to keep moving — if I stop, I get tired.
- ☐ Feeling overwhelmed by all that needs to be done
- ☐ It takes all my energy to do what I have to — there's none left over for anything or anyone else

FACTORS LEADING TO ADRENAL FATIGUE

White sugar and white flour products	Stimulants
Lack of relaxation	Negative thinking
Smoking	Oral contraceptives
Antacids	Non-prescription drug use
Devitalized food	Psychological stress
Unfulfilling employment	Persistent fears
Unfulfilling relationships	Emotional stress
Surgery	Lack of sleep
Unhealthy diet filled with junk food	Inability to address your feelings/denial
Consuming trans fats and/or rancid fats	Infection, acute or chronic
Financial stress	Persistent negative stressors
Sedentary lifestyle	Fun or enjoyment deprivation
Excessive exercise	Allergies
Death of a loved one	Caffeine
Alcoholism	Prescription drug use
Toxins	Marital stress
Hormonal imbalances	Repeated traumas
Conventional hormone replacement therapy	Workaholic

I would suggest you look over the two assessments and see how many symptoms you recognize in your own life. If you're experiencing sexual challenges and your overall personal health score is low, you should commit to making some changes. It will require discipline and new habit patterns. Many of the changes are actually counter-cultural in our fast-paced world, but your physical and sexual health is worth the effort! Start slowly by choosing a few new habits. As you are successful and your health starts to improve, it will give you great satisfaction and the motivation to do even more for your body and your sex life.

THE SYMPATHETIC AND PARASYMPATHETIC NERVOUS SYSTEMS

We've touched on the two significant players for favorable hormonal health, the sympathetic and parasympathetic nervous systems. It will be helpful for you to know if your body is sympathetic or parasympathetic dominant. (Most people become parasympathetic dominant after their adrenal glands have become exhausted.)

The autonomic nervous system is a principal regulator of body function. It's composed of the sympathetic and parasympathetic systems. The sympathetic system is designed for fight or flight and thus favors the muscular system and the body's ability to respond physically with increased performance in threatening situations. Its balancing counterpart, the parasympathetic nervous system, is designed for promoting digestion, keeping the mucus membranes moist, (think vaginal lubrication!) and promoting day-to-day management of the internal workings of the body.

Sympathetic types tend to have high energy, aggressive personalities, weak digestion, dry skin (there's that vaginal lubrication component again!) and excellent concentration. They tend to be tall, thin, have narrow shoulders, wider hips and are commonly underweight. They build muscle easily and tend to crave carbohydrates. They are prone to osteoporosis, infections, angina, heart disease, cancer, acute arthritis, diabetes, gall bladder attacks, ulcers, glaucoma and gingivitis (inflamed gums).

Excessive sympathetic responses fatigue the pituitary, thyroid, adrenals and/or the ovaries and testes (this is described in more detail in the Hormone Chapter). I would like to mention that there is no real significant anatomical or nervous tissue component difference between the two systems; the difference is the biochemicals that are involved.

Parasympathetic types tend to be slow, deliberate, and cautious about their feelings. They are usually emotionally stable and able to make friends easily. They sometimes have low motivation, a tendency for allergies and asthma, low blood sugar, skin problems, and poor concentration. They are generally wider built, with broad shoulders and good strength and endurance. Often their pupils are constricted, the membranes of the mouth and nose are moist with excess saliva/mucus, their heart rate is slow, and their blood pressure is low.

Parasympathetic dominance promotes osteoarthritis and calcification of soft tissues, as with cataracts, kidney stones, calcific bursitis, heel and bone spurs, hardening of the arteries and heart valves. From the standpoint of whole-body health, it is important to have balance in the autonomic nervous system. This allows for optimal metabolism and digestion. The glands involved in function of the parasympathetic nervous system include the pituitary, thyroid and adrenal tissues. It's important to note that the parasympathetic nervous system promotes digestion and is also responsible for relaxation and sleep.

A healthy person is able to appropriately engage the para-sympathetic and the sympathetic nervous systems at the necessary times with great benefit to body, mind and spirit. The parasympathetic and sympathetic nervous systems must be regulated to the precise degree in the correct timing, reacting to the circumstance at hand. In certain situations an individual may need to be nearly 100 percent parasympathetic (while eating dinner); at others, 40 percent parasympathetic and 60 percent sympathetic (drinking water while taking a walk with your spouse). And less often, 100 percent sympathetic (immediately following a natural disaster). Environmental circumstances determine the needed percentages. When both systems are working in correct balance, they are a marvel! When one or the other becomes dominant, the nervous system becomes a hindrance rather than a help in accomplishing daily tasks.

If, as you read this, you are becoming more determined to engage or disengage your sympathetic or parasympathetic systems through willpower, think again. The balance between them is an *unconscious* act that functions more perfectly only when you make *conscious* choices toward good health.

Here is a simple screen to determine which category you fall into: Look over the following groups of symptoms and mark the ones that describe you. You may recognize yourself in both groups but generally score higher in one or the other.

PERSONAL HEALTH ASSESSMENT

Sympathetic Dominant		
☐ Acid foods upset	☐ High gag reflex	☐ Reduced appetite
☐ Often feel chilled	☐ Unable to relax; startles easily	☐ Frequent cold sweats
☐ "Lump" in throat	☐ Extremities cold, clammy	☐ Fever easily raised
☐ Dry mouth, eyes, nose	☐ Irritated by strong light	☐ Neuralgia-like pains
☐ Pulse quickens after meal	☐ Urine amount reduced	☐ Staring, blinks little
☐ Nervous tension, unable to calm oneself	☐ Heart pounds after retiring	☐ Frequent sour stomach

Parasympathetic Dominant		
☐ Joint stiffness after rising	☐ Always seems hungry; feels "lightheaded" often	☐ Difficulty swallowing
☐ Muscle, leg, toe cramps at night	☐ Rapid Digestion	☐ Constipation, diarrhea alternating
☐ Nervous stomach, cramps	☐ Frequent vomiting	☐ Slow starter
☐ Eyes or nose watery	☐ Frequent hoarseness	☐ Not easily chilled
☐ Eyes blink often	☐ Irregular breathing	☐ Perspire easily
☐ Eyelids swollen, puffy	☐ Pulse slow; feels "irregular"	☐ Poor circulation Sensitive to cold
☐ Indigestion soon after meals	☐ Little gag reflex	☐ Subject to colds, asthma, bronchitis

If you marked several in the first list you would tend to be sympathetic dominant. Specific treatments determined by a qualified healthcare provider may be helpful depending on the specific symptoms you're experiencing.

Those who score high in the second group of symptoms tend to be parasympathetic dominant individuals. From my clinical observation, these patients were formerly sympathetic dominant, but they fed their cravings and body signals with stimulants, such as caffeine and sugar, leading to adrenal exhaustion and many of the symptoms in the Sympathetic Dominance Table. The more symptoms an individual checks in the assessment above, the more of an autonomic imbalance they tend to have. I've found this to be the case regardless of which group they fall into. Eventually, they'll experience multiple symptoms from *both* groups as their nervous system function degrades more and more over time.

The parasympathetic nervous systemactivity — including vaginal lubrication —is overridden and may actually shut down, leaving this frustrated woman with yet *another* stressful symptom: vaginal dryness. The same process is true for persistently stressed men resulting in difficulty achieving and maintaining erections.

Most patients experiencing the sexual dysfunction rampant in our fast-paced culture fall into the sympathetic dominant nervous system category. When a woman, for example, is chronically stressed by her normal day-to-day activities, the constant adrenal excitation creates fatigue. Instead of recognizing the demands she is placing on her body and taking appropriate actions to reduce stress, many reach for artificial stimulants mentioned above such as sugar and caffeine-laden soda and energy drinks to get through the day. These temporarily avert physical exhaustion but continue to fuel sympathetic dominance. The parasympathetic nervous system activity —

including vaginal lubrication — is overridden and may actually shut down, leaving this frustrated woman with yet *another* stressful symptom: vaginal dryness. The same process is true for persistently stressed men resulting in difficulty achieving and maintaining erections. Stress results in sympathetic dominance, the adrenal excitation creates fatigue, and he reaches for artificial stimulants leading to continued sympathetic dominance. At the end of a stress-filled day, this couple goes to make love with each other and the whole vicious cycle has robbed their bodies of the ability to have spontaneous, enjoyable sex — the one thing that has the potential to bring the most relaxation and pleasure to their day!

Medication can treat both of these symptoms, but it adds a number of sobering side effects to an already fatigued body. Medication also ignores the other body alert signals of autonomic nervous system imbalance. Equally troubling is the prospect of taking medication to correct *every* symptom experienced; imagine what a potentially fatal drug cocktail that would look like! No, treatment does not have to be as complicated as a medicine cabinet that resembles the local drugstore. You have the power to make small changes that will return your body to the wonderfully balanced state God intended. Of course, it's best to have the assistance of a knowledgeable health care provider as you take steps toward health and wholeness.

If you checked multiple boxes on the symptom list and suspect that your adrenal gland function is compromised, now is the time to make some changes. We learned in the first paragraph of this chapter that your body is a complex, *interdependent* network of systems whose functions impact each other in multiple ways. This is wonderful news, because small changes will have a *profound* impact throughout your whole body, including empowering it for enduring *lovemaking*! As you care for your body, it will pay you back with great health, great energy, great enjoyment, and great sex.

JUST TELL ME WHAT TO DO

❑ A true key to long-term adrenal health is adequate rest. Make whatever changes are necessary in your schedule to assure eight hours of sleep each night. Limit TV and computer time before bed to allow your mind and body time to relax without stimulation. Sleep in a cool, dark room; cover the small lights from your alarm clock and appliances. If you are experiencing adrenal exhaustion, make arrangements that allow you to sleep until between 7 and 9am each morning.

❑ Gymnema is an excellent herb that reduces the taste for sweet items; take one to three daily.

❑ Add more protein to your diet. Protein helps stabilize the rate your body burns energy and eliminates the extreme highs and lows that sugar induces. If you are consuming large amounts of nutritionally empty carbohydrates, your system will actually burn *muscle* to get the energy it needs to function. Limit protein to three to five ounces per serving so you do not get a compensatory insulin release, which can start a cascade of cravings for sweets.

❑ Avoid sweet fruits, especially bananas, raisins and grapes. Eat veggies as a snack with some nuts such as almonds, walnuts and sunflower seeds.

❑ If you crave salt (a common adrenal fatigue symptom), consume Celtic Sea Salt®.

❑ Ladies, I do not suggest the long-term use of topical progesterone cream because it literally tricks the feedback mechanisms into interpreting that your hormone levels are normal. Progesterone cream can be used for a very short time period if you're experiencing relentless heavy menstrual flow that is not responding to care. Still, your long-term plan should be reaching a level of health that enables your body to create the progesterone it needs.

❑ I'd also advise you to avoid supplementing DHEA, which can upset the delicate balance of hormones in your body. Instead, seek out a skilled healthcare provider to help you manage adrenal fatigue.

❑ Consume Vitamin C-sourced foods. A delicious choice and one that is available year round is a mixed green salad with Vitamin C-rich red, yellow and orange bell peppers. Vitamin C is an integral component of adrenal health. I do not encourage citrus because it tends to create an alkaline pH, commonly observed in females over 40 resulting in fibromyalgia.

❑ Those with low blood pressure should consider using a whole food B complex vitamin supplement. Again, you should consult an experienced health care provider during treatment.

❑ Get a hair analysis to determine your adrenal health. This test will often reveal decreased sodium and potassium and increased aluminum when a patient has stressed adrenal function. The test also determines other mineral levels and is useful in creating a treatment program.

❑ Complete saliva hormone testing to get a baseline of your endocrine and hormone systems' function. Free hormones are measured in saliva testing; protein-bound hormones in serum testing. Go to www.druglessdoctor.com for details.

13

Change Your Filter for Better Performance

As you read this book we hope you're fully grasping what a wonderful and complex machine your body is. You're like a mega computer system made up of trillions of cells all working together for the good of the whole. 1 Corinthians 12:12-26 teaches that the body is a unit made up of many parts, none of which is greater than any other. I'm reminded of this remarkable concept as I work with my patients each day. When one part suffers it affects the function of the whole, and when one part is brought to health the rest of the body benefits as well.

Your liver is an amazing organ, responsible for hundreds of functions which involve your sex life. When the liver is overworked there is commonly an abundance of unprocessed natural and synthetic estrogen. As we will discuss below, hormonal imbalances are responsible for breast tenderness and heavy menses in women. Estrogen can also accumulate in men, creating prostate challenges including prostate enlargement. In addition, the liver is involved in storing blood and vitamins, processing hormones, releasing blood sugar and protein, destroying unwanted organisms, creating bile for fat metabolism, eliminating unwanted consumed and cellular debris and much more. When you eat toxic, processed foods, your liver rearranges the chemical structures and releases residual by-products through urine, sweat, your breath and the colon.

There's a process that occurs in the liver called the P450 system which neutralizes medications and toxic substances by binding them to proteins and sulfur and then flushing them from the body. When liver function is compromised the normal filtering process decreases, commonly resulting in degenerative conditions including cancer and arthritis. Imagine driving through an expanding community with a limited sewer system. You'd likely smell the backup of sewage. Decreased liver function can be recognized in much the same way: foul breath, rank-smelling stool, skin rashes and skin tags (these are usually brown flarings off your skin).

An overworked liver places additional stress on the kidneys, which also aid in detoxification and can be considered the liver's "helper." Symptoms of kidney stress include high blood pressure, swollen legs and general swelling of the body. Low thyroid function and the constipation may result in additional stress on the liver.

Years of treating patients and studying texts have brought me to a rather curious conclusion about the liver: it's an organ that's effected by emotions. Have you recognized more road rage over the last few years as I have? You may have even noticed that those same people who are driving recklessly have a burger and fries in their hand as they shake their fist at you! They're eating fast and furiously while honking the horn and yelling at everyone around them. It comes with no surprise that studies show eating in a distressed state creates digestion problems and liver distress. In these conditions, your liver is literally being jammed by your emotions while simultaneously attempting to rid your body of toxic processed foods. According to Eastern medical philosophy, anger is associated with the liver. These cultures also associate the liver with romantic occasions like engagements and weddings much like Americans exchange heart-shaped cards on Valentines' Day. Love creates enormous emotions in the body, and the combination of love and a passionate, monogamous marriage create the perfect environment for optimum liver function.

You can see what a vital service the liver performs, including storing the fat-soluble vitamins A, D, E and K which support sexual functions. Striving for peak liver function should be one of your daily goals.

I encourage you to become more aware of what you put in (and on) your body and its effect on your liver. Foods like diet soft drinks, alcohol and prescription medications create liver distress. Your liver needs to clear those burdensome chemical toxins found in conventional non-organic food so they don't hinder cellular function. Your diet should be based on fresh organic whole foods which require very little assistance from the liver; every bite of over-processed, nutrient-empty food needs to be neutralized and eliminated by your liver detoxification system. Why make your liver's job even harder by feeding it toxins?

Start each day with a glass of warm water and a wedge of washed organic lemon. Let the lemon soak in the water a few minutes, then drink the liquid and eat the lemon pulp, discarding the rind. This technique is a great way to stimulate liver function and digestion. I also recommend eating at least half of a red apple daily[1], as well as one-third cup of fresh, organic beets, baked or raw and grated. Add at least five small baby carrots or a medium whole carrot each day to consume what I call "Dr. Bob's ABCs." These power foods will help stimulate normal liver function.

---

1   Avoid green apples, as they slow digestion.

The skin is a report card on how your liver is performing. You may have suffered from acne when you were a teenager, and it's not uncommon for adults to have acne breakouts through their thirties.[2] Your skin is actually one of the largest organs in the body and is used to rid the body of unwanted substances. In my experience, skin challenges can almost always be traced to an overworked liver handling toxic food, beverages and even over-the-counter and prescription medications. Proper liver maintenance will eventually ease skin flare-ups, though it may continue to take several months and possibly even years for your complexion to become fully clear.

The liver is a component in the stabilization of blood sugar by signaling cells to either store excess glucose or release it for fuel. Eating a diet high in sugar upsets this balance. In addition, the liver works with the pancreas during digestion. The pancreas releases insulin and enzymes for metabolism. Sluggish liver function decreases bile production, leading to digestive distress and impaired fat and sugar metabolism. Another reason a diet high in sugar and processed foods is destructive is because these nutrient-deficient products place incredible strain on the liver and pancreas and greatly increase the incidence of diabetes. Men have an added incentive to do everything possible to avoid this disease as diabetics historically suffer from erectile dysfunction in all its forms.

I'd like to recommend a treatment to facilitate liver cleansing that can be used in the comfort of your own home. I encourage my patients (both male and female) to incorporate the highly effective Castor Oil Pack into their weekly routine. While this may seem like an exotic approach to detoxification and liver

---

2   A common cause of adult-onset acne is the hormones in birth control pills, which will be discussed in more detail below.

efficiency, in reality it's a low budget, low tech method to assist in cleansing. You can read more about castor oil and its uses in the Castor Oil Appendix 4.

Decreased liver function can commonly be associated with high blood pressure and depression. Emotions do have the ability to affect organ function! I've discovered through experience that the right fat choices have everything to do with behavioral and emotional health. I supplement patients who are depressed with organic high lignan Omega 3 flax oil. The flax oil provides the precursor nutrients needed for DHA in the brain; this fatty acid is one of the many nutrients required for optimal brain health. A happy brain controls a happy body, and a happy body is capable of giving and receiving sensational sexual pleasure!

Do you still have your gall bladder? Over one-half million gall bladders are removed every year in America through cholecystectomy surgery. Your gall bladder stores bile, which acts like a dish detergent that breaks apart the fats you eat and keeps them from accumulating on blood vessel walls and the lining of organs. When your gall bladder is removed, you lose this sack of stored bile and have no backup source for those times when more fat needs to be processed. Decreased bile levels lead to an accumulation of fat in the colon, resulting in an anaerobic (decreased oxygen) environment that is hospitable to cancer. You often hear that eating "saturated fat" causes colon cancer; in reality, cancer patients often have deeper challenges in the form of decreased bile output due to compromised liver function. If you've had your gall bladder removed, you should add a whole food bile salt to your diet indefinitely to remain healthy and combat cancer and heart disease.

TOXIC OVERLOAD

We are bombarded by man made synthetic compounds daily. I have mentioned that these substances must be cleared by the liver for you to thrive physically. I am strongly encouraging you to become very perceptive of your environment and what you are putting in and on your body. We are at a point in our society where you can not stay passive any more about chemical exposure: you must become knowledgeable and proactive. Label reading is critical, but it may all not be factual. "Even products marketed as "natural" can come packed with hormone disrupters, carcinogens, toxic-by products, and heavy metals. In fact, the average woman applies more than 150 chemicals through her skin care daily" according to Lindsey Galloway and Elizabeth Marglin in a recent article in Natural Solutions, in an article title "Beauty With a Conscience." It is very important for you to become enlightened on what products are safe. I would suggest you may want to search the American Cancer Society's web page on products that are carcinogenic.

Let's take it up one more very serious step; the water you are choosing to drink may be hazardous to your health. Wow, that was a bold statement. The municipal drinking water in America has deteriorated exponentially as of late and unfortunately very few appear to be aware of the significance. Some time ago a report was released about pharmaceutical trace residues being detected in and around municipalities. In a recent article titled, "Discarded Drugs Affect More Drinking Water" released by The Associated Press, said that up to 46 million Americans are being affected by pharmaceuticals in the drinking water. The list of items found in the water include a cholesterol and nicotine derivative, many communities have found and anti-convulsant carbamazepine. Other communities have detected other pharmaceuticals including a tranquilizer and a hormone. Let me tell you, do not be duped by your community officials and manufacturers of these compounds that they are at safe levels. Insist that your local community test the water that is produced by the filtration plant. I would also suggest you may want to purchase a water purifier for your home.

Processing estrogen is another of the liver's functions, and B vitamins are a critical component in this process. Once again, sugar and stress are major culprits that deplete the body of B vitamins. Now you can see why many people are unknowingly sabotaging liver function. The chart below lists common signs of B deficiencies; how many symptoms are you experiencing?

☐ Apprehension	☐ Depression	☐ Nervousness
☐ Irritability	☐ Noise sensitivity	☐ Headache
☐ Morbid fears	☐ Acoustic hallucinations	☐ Insomnia
☐ Hypochondrea	☐ Tendency to cry without reason	☐ Anxiety
☐ Forgetfulness	☐ Feelings of dread	☐ Anorexia
☐ Indigestion	☐ Weakness	☐ Distraction
☐ Poor appetite	☐ Fatigue	☐ Confusion
☐ Craving for sweets	☐ Neuralgia	☐ Dizziness

If you marked five or more boxes you should evaluate your diet to determine what foods are overworking your liver and causing the symptoms of estrogen overload. These symptoms can usually be improved with proper whole food B vitamin supplementation.

Unfortunately, I see many women as young as thirty-five to forty who are struggling with the effects of increased estrogen levels. This hormone creates cellular proliferation (growth) in the body and needs to be balanced by progesterone.[3] The delicate balance of these hormones is upset by stress and an unhealthy diet and lifestyle, leading to estrogen dominance and saturation.

---

3   See the Adrenal Gland Chapter for a detailed discussion of hormone balance.

ESTROGEN OVERLOAD

One of the largest challenges I've discovered affecting both men and women of all ages is the magnitude of xenohormones or synthetic estrogens ingested from the environment. These hormones are commonly found in polycarbonate, one of the plastics carrying the recycling Number 7 symbol. The plastic is clear, tough and lightweight, making it ideal for everything from bulletproof glass to water bottles, sippy cups, dental sealants, plastic eating utensils and food storage containers. The BPA in polycarbonates is also found in the epoxy resins lining the inside of food and beverage cans, which leak in small amounts into the food or water in the containers. In fact, the list of items containing xenohormones is nearly endless, including the dust in our homes and our air and water!

What worries some scientists is that BPA is an estrogenic "mimic," activating the same receptors in the body as estrogen does. In fact, BPA was first studied in the 1930s as a synthetic estrogen for women.

"BPA is the largest-volume endocrine-disrupting chemical in commerce," says BPA critic Frederick Vom Saul, a biologist at the University of Missouri, Worldwide. More than six million pounds of BPA are manufactured every year and Vom Saul is convinced that BPA causes a host of problems including breast and prostate cancer.[4]

You and your entire family are continuously and relentlessly bombarded with BPA in the form of canned foods, car exhaust, fingernail polish, aerosol sprays, paints, noxious vapor compounds released from carpets, wall paper, and magazine ink, just to name a few. The physical results of exposure and resulting liver congestion include spider veins, hemorrhoids, varicose

---

4   Nutrition Action, Center for Science in the Public Interest, April 2008.

veins, skin tags on the neck, face and body, and the elusive cherry hemangiomas. The sexual consequences are even more sobering: tender breasts and heavy menses in women, prostate swelling and cancer in men, accelerated secondary sexual characteristics in children, increased sexual appetites in young girls and effeminate tendencies in boys. It's time to evaluate what can be done to protect you and your family from toxic exposure.

How to Minimize Your Exposure to BPA

> Avoid plastic containers made of polycarbonate. (Any bottle or container made of polycarbonate that has the recycling Number 7 on the bottom.) Be aware that Number 7 can also appear on plastics not containing BPA.

> When possible, prepare or store food – especially hot foods and liquids – in glass, porcelain, or stainless steel dishes or containers.

> If you have polycarbonate plastic containers, don't microwave them. The plastic is more likely to break down and release BPA when it's repeatedly heated at high temperatures.

> Don't wash polycarbonate containers in the dishwasher. The detergent may break down the plastic, resulting in the release of BPA.

> Use glass infant formula bottles or those free of BPA plastic. BornFree (newbornfree.com) is one of the first companies manufacturing them. This is very important for the health of your children.

> When possible, replace canned foods with those that are fresh, frozen or packaged in aseptic (shelf stable) boxes. Be mindful and look for "BPA Free" labels.

> Currently, a possible alternative to polycarbonate is polyethelene terephthalate (PETE), which is marked with the recycling Number 1 symbol.

➤ Avoid older versions of Delton dental sealant. Dental sealants are plastic resins a dentist bonds into the grooves of the chewing surface of teeth to help prevent cavities.

The liver is just one organ in an amazingly complex machine, but it's a very critical one! Decreased function results in symptoms affecting almost every system in the body. The good news is that choices made to improve liver health ultimately benefit every other part as well, *including* sexual function. Start making wise decisions today and experience all that God intended in your body *and your bedroom* through optimal liver function!

JUST TELL ME WHAT TO DO

❑ Avoid processed foods, which stress the liver. Instead, eat organic fresh, lightly steamed, raw or sautéed whole foods.

❑ Avoid items which may create an extra burden on liver function: medications, alcohol, soft drinks and artificial sweeteners or preservatives.

❑ Consume only organic meat products to avoid estrogen-fed animal tissue. Look at the label where your food originated. It is now the law in the U.S. to state the country of origin for food items.

❑ Minimize your exposure to PBA by avoiding canned foods. Start drinking water from glass containers instead of plastic bottles.

❑ Eat Dr. Bob's ABCs: ½ of a red apple, one third cup of beets and four or five baby carrots daily.

❑ Avoid the constipation that leads to liver distress by drinking more water and eating whole foods.

❑ Follow the castor oil pack routine as a great therapeutic treatment to improve liver function.

Natural Solutions, October 2008. Lindsey Galloway and Elizabeth Marglin "Beauty With a Conscience."

The Chronicle Telegram. Friday September 12th. AP "Discarded Drugs Affect More Drinking Water" author, Martha Mendoza

14
Turning Up the Heat

"**C**old hands, warm heart" is an old cliché, but having cold hands can be an awkward warning sign of thyroid problems. The thyroid gland is located in the middle of the throat and is an important component of the endocrine system. It has many roles, including regulating body temperature and ensuring that you will have warm hands *and* a warm heart! The thyroid regulates metabolism (including bowel and colon function) and also works closely with the adrenal glands to provide energy. Sexual desire and ability are closely related to and affected by thyroid function.

In our fast-paced society, it's not uncommon for both men and women to experience thyroid and adrenal gland exhaustion, resulting in decreased energy and lowered sexual desire. Low thyroid function is one of the most common diagnoses among new patients who come to me seeking natural treatment for health issues. They feel out-of-control and overwhelmed and few consider that their problems may be caused by decreased thyroid function. Many are taking Synthroid, a common prescription medication for low thyroid activity and are beginning to question its validity in the face of more natural treatment methods. Others are being pressured to start thyroid medication and are hesitant to do so due to negative side effects. Look over the following list of symptoms and see if you recognize any in your own life:

COMMON LOW THYROID BODY SIGNALS

➢ Hot flashes

➢ Constipation

➢ Emotional distress

➢ Low progesterone-estrogen levels

➢ Morning headaches that wear off as the day progresses

➢ Feeling chilled in the morning

➢ Colds hands and feet

➢ High cholesterol

➢ Coarse hair that falls out

➢ Widely-spaced teeth

➢ Thinning hair

➢ Nighttime urination

➢ Fatigue

➢ Obesity

➢ Thinning of the outer eyebrows

➢ Yellow teeth

HOT FLASHES, FEELING CHILLED, COLD EXTREMITIES

The thyroid acts like a thermostat to regulate body temperature. Many patients complain of being chilled in the fall and winter. If you find yourself wearing winter pajamas all year 'round, your thyroid may be suspect. This chronic condition may impact sexual intimacy if one partner is always cold and reluctant to undress for the event. You can always turn up the heat in your bedroom, but treating the condition is simple and will result in even greater benefits! Having a healthy and regulated body temperature offers you both the wonderful opportunity to slip into bed without pajamas and still feel warm. And who knows what that might lead to?!

If you experience feeling chilled and cold hands and feet you may want to limit your intake of cruciferous foods, including broccoli, cauliflower, and cabbage. For the general public these are excellent sources of nutrients and fiber, but I've found they sometimes impair thyroid function and should be avoided at least for a while. Once body temperature is regulated, you may add them back into your diet, either steaming or sautéing the vegetables. It's not necessary to eat them raw as some health journals suggest, and cooking them slightly might actually deter some of the digestive challenges they often present. Soy products should be avoided since they are antagonistic to thyroid function. To ensure proper fiber in your diet during this time, consume green beans, zucchini, peppers, asparagus, and steamed carrots. Deb and I enjoy a mixed green salad for lunch almost every day, avoiding iceberg lettuce which has little if any nutritional value.

A more significant thyroid difficulty affects women in the form of dreaded hot flashes. As the thyroid grows stressed and exhausted, it loses the ability to regulate body temperature and results in the heater always set to "On." I've discovered this is often caused by a lack of iodine in the diet, which is discussed in more detail further in this chapter. Toxins such as bromine, fluorine and chlorine compete with iodine, further impairing thyroid function. Excessive intake of processed foods full of partially hydrogenated fat (trans fat) impedes liver function, in turn limiting the hormones the thyroid needs to regulate temperature.[1] It's been my experience that hot flashes are one of the leading reasons women seek natural health care, along with heavy menstrual flow.

---

1   You can read more about natural methods for hormonal balance in *Dr. Bob's Drugless Guide to Balancing Female Hormones*.

CONSTIPATION

Because the thyroid has an impact on bowel and colon activity, its impairment often results in constipation. Many people, especially women, choose to treat constipation with laxatives. While laxatives may work temporarily, it's easy to become dependent on them for bowel movements and continue ignoring your body's cry for healthy habits. The correct natural method to treat this condition is by increasing water and fiber consumption. I often encourage my patients to allow time for rest and relaxation in the morning, which generally leads to a bowel movement. Constipation can also become a significant but largely ignored deterrent to sexual activity. The competition between stool and the penis for the limited space in the pelvic cavity may cause women to feel full and uncomfortable.

EMOTIONAL DISTRESS

Many people seeking psychiatric treatment for emotional issues are often suffering from impaired thyroid function. Stress has an incredibly large impact on the thyroid and adrenal glands, causing fatigue and anxiety.

I've actually treated patients who experienced panic attacks as their weddings approached – both brides *and* grooms! One patient ended up in the emergency room three days before the wedding. After consulting them I determined the anxiety attack was in response to an overdose of sugar. This sweet culprit robs the body of nutrients needed for enzyme and hormone function. (I always felt kind of bad for this couple. If the wedding itself was so stressful, I can't imagine what the rest of the marriage will be like....)

If you have chronic emotional distress, you should have a proper thyroid assessment by an experienced health care professional familiar with endocrine function and natural treatment of such. I see more and more young patients, especially women, who are currently taking two different prescription antidepressants. This is a sobering trend among young people who are being medicated and overmedicated at a crucial time in their lives as they are starting careers, marriages and families. They would be better served by a thyroid malfunction diagnosis and natural treatment of their symptoms rather than masking the problem with prescription drugs. If you are currently taking any medications for emotional distress issues, you should not discontinue them until talking with your doctor. Tyrosine and iodine combine to create thyroid hormone. Tyrosine is an amino acid that is clinically proven to aid in the treatment of depression. Adding tyrosine to my patients' treatment has consistently benefited those dealing with emotional challenges.

I don't intend to deliberately pinpoint women in a discussion of emotional distress, but I do treat far more women than men for depression and depression-related syndromes. I believe this is simply based on the fact that women have a larger puzzle of hormones (including iodine deficiencies) in their endocrine balance sheet then men do. Men primarily need iodine for thyroid and testes/prostate function, while women need it for proper function of all their hormones and for the thyroid, breasts and ovaries. It still remains true, however, that the health of every cell in both men and women is impacted by iodine.

Other possible factors in depression include insufficient Omega 3 oils, lack of minerals and low supply of B vitamins. Many doctors are quick to prescribe medication, but they come with the unfortunate side effect of diminished sexual appetite. Once again, the symptoms are treated, the cause is masked, and negative side effects wreak their own havoc on the body and the marriage. Increasing thyroid function with natural methods is so simple and successful – I don't know why anyone wouldn't want to give it a try when the benefits are so quickly experienced.

LOW PROGESTERONE-ESTROGEN LEVELS

My experience has shown that patients who are deficient in iodine are often lacking in progesterone. Women who are lacking iodine have compromised ovaries and an inadequate supply of nutrients for the production of estrogen-balancing progesterone.

MANAGING A MORNING HEADACHE

Headaches in the morning can be a real...PAIN! They certainly don't increase the incidence of quick morning sexual romps, a time of day when many men wake up with erections that could be utilized. When I treat a patient who wakes up with morning headaches, I always ask first what they ate before going to sleep. The most common answer is something full of sugar, even a food as seemingly harmless as a sweet dried fruit. During the night, the thyroid and adrenal processing of sugar is decreased, resulting in increased blood sugar and voila! — a morning headache. When men come to me asking about their spouse's morning headaches, it generally means they aren't getting any morning action! Simply cutting out sugar often puts a smile on the faces of husband and wife alike.

HIGH CHOLESTEROL

Cholesterol elevates in patients with low thyroid function. Cholesterol-lowering medications often put added strain on the liver, and an overworked liver suppresses libido. If you suspect reduced liver function with elevated cholesterol, add beets to your diet. Cholesterol attaches to the beet fiber and is escorted out of the body with your bowel movement. (You should eat beets rather than juicing them for purposes of cholesterol management.)

FATIGUE

The thyroid's role in energy is like the gas pedal on a car. No gas, no energy, no sex.[2] While fatigue can occur at any age, I especially see couples over forty suffering from this condition.

OBESITY

There are many reasons why people struggle with obesity; the most obvious is consuming more calories then you are burning each day. However, many doctors overlook the fact that patients who are overweight tend to have an iodine deficiency due to poor diet choices and antagonistic challenges from bromine, fluorine and chlorine. A fully functioning thyroid maintains normal metabolism, reducing the storage of those extra calories. Patients with low thyroid function generally lose weight once thyroid stabilization occurs.

COARSE HAIR THAT FALLS OUT, THINNING OF THE HAIR AND EYEBROWS, WIDELY-SPACED AND/OR YELLOW TEETH

Minerals affect thyroid gland productivity. When the thyroid is stressed or does not receive adequate nutritional building blocks, mineral absorption decreases. The results vary, from changes in hair texture, thinning of hair on the head and eyebrows, to changes in teeth placement. Yellowed teeth are also common in patients with a sluggish thyroid as calcium uptake is impaired and teeth become discolored.

THE ROLE OF IODINE IN THYROID FUNCTION

Iodine is one of the major components the thyroid uses to create thyroid hormone; unfortunately, the amount of iodine consumed in the U.S. is largely inadequate. If you believe you're getting

---

2   Refer to the "Not Tonight! I'm Too Tired!" chapter for a detailed
      discussion of energy levels.

iodine in table salt, think again. The iodized salt purchased at conventional grocery stores generally contains aluminum and dextrose for anti-caking purposes and I don't encourage its use. Sodium chloride (table salt) can actually create challenges with normal thyroid function. Instead, my clients switch to hand-harvested Celtic Sea Salt®. It's a great source of easily-assimilated minerals including iodine.

I also want you to be aware of some anti-thyroid nutrients that can interfere with the normal receptor sites for iodine. As I mentioned above, these include bromine, fluorine and chlorine. Bromine replaced iodine as a conditioner in bread in the early 1960's. Commercial white bread products, consumed in great quantities in America, can actually create thyroid distress. Bromine is found in certain beverages including soda and sports drinks and is an ingredient in some anti-depressants. The irony is sobering: that psycho-active medications commonly used to treat depression can actually *promote* it as bromine interferes with iodine metabolism.

Fluorine is put in most municipalities' water supplies and is also a common oral application at well-meaning dental offices. Deb and I personally do not drink tap water nor do we receive fluoride treatments, and we haven't had a cavity in decades. The same is true for both of our sons who were born in the 1980s.

Chlorine is a little known but very common anti-iodine nutrient. If you use a dishwasher detergent that contains this toxic chemical and happen to breathe it in, you're getting your share of chlorine. The same is true of the steam you inhale while taking a shower in chlorinated water. For this reason, I encourage the use of chlorine-free dishwasher soap as well as the installation of a de-chlorinating showerhead. You should also limit the amount of time spent in hot tubs and swimming pools. We've seen patients who suffer from chronic leg cramps as a result of swimming and exercising in bromine- and chlorine-saturated pools. Splenda®, which is sourced from sugar, also stresses the thyroid due to the chlorine in its composition.

I can't overstate the vital role iodine plays in the production of hormones affecting sexuality. Without it, a woman's ovaries are unable to produce sufficient amounts of progesterone, the hormone that balances estrogen levels in women. Imbalance results in estrogen dominance or saturation and can lead to tender breasts and heavy, painful menstruation. Men's PSA prostate assessment levels lower when their diet is supplemented with adequate iodine and they are monitored by the urine iodine loading test.

The Barnes Thyroid armpit test is a simple way to screen if your thyroid is possibly not functioning as it should. Place a shaken down or battery-operated thermometer by your bedside some evening. The next morning, upon waking, place the stem of thermometer in your armpit for ten minutes. (This should be done even before getting out of bed and going to the bathroom.) The temperature reading should be 97.8 F or higher; if it's lower, you should focus on adding a source of iodine to your diet.[3] This can be in the form of kelp, sea vegetables, ocean seafood or Celtic Sea Salt®. Repeat this simple self assessment at least monthly while supplementing with iodine-based foods. If your temperature hasn't changed, seek a natural health care provider who has experience treating thyroid conditions with appropriate supplementation and diet modifications. Mineral tissue hair analysis may also be an important step in the diagnosis of a thyroid-related problem.

---

3   A low morning body temperature reading may also be caused by inadequate function of the pituitary, liver and adrenal glands. See the Hormone chapter for more information on treatment.

Your healthcare provider may check your TSH, T3 and T4 levels to determine if thyroid hormone levels are sufficient. Low levels of T3 and T4 often suggest a deficiency of both tyrosine and iodine. The treatment for high TSH often includes a form of cell therapy with an animal tissue source of thyroid DNA. A low TSH reading may suggest the pituitary gland is in need of some assistance. Occasionally these tests come back with normal levels even though a patient is experiencing all the common symptoms of thyroid malfunction such as cold extremities, constipation and high cholesterol. If the tests are within normal range and you suspect your thyroid is the cause, seek a health care provider who is open to natural forms of treatment.

A diet full of nutrients that impact thyroid health includes flax oil, beets, plenty of protein, sea vegetables and deep ocean fish. Fruits should be limited. You may not notice changes in your thyroid tests for up to two years upon initiating a natural protocol, but you would be wise to pursue a natural treatment as thyroid medication does not cure the problem nor assist the body in calcium metabolism.

JUST TELL ME WHAT TO DO

❑ Browse the symptom list and choose one or two areas of thyroid health that can be improved. If you have multiple symptoms, commit to making at least one diet or lifestyle change each week.

❑ Have your urine iodine levels assessed and supplement accordingly.

❑ Avoid exposure to bromine, fluorine and chlorine. Obtain a water purifier and a shower de-chlorinator.

❑ Complete the armpit temperature test. If the level is below 97.8°F you may want to seek treatment from an experienced natural healthcare provider and have a TSH, T3 and T4 test.

❑ Avoid soy and other foods that deplete iodine.

15

Is it Time for a Pause?

Mention the word "menopause" in a crowd of women and you're sure to get a pretty strong reaction. Now that sexuality has been brought out into public view, everyone has heard the horror stories and jokes that go along with this "second change of life."

The medical definition of menopause is much simpler than you probably realize: "The period of permanent cessation of menstruation, usually occurring between the ages of 45 and 55." That's all — no tales of hot flashes, night sweats and vaginal dryness. Could menopause really be that simple? Yes!

Menopause is a natural decrease in estrogen levels that stops the menstrual cycle, keeping a woman from conceiving and carrying a child.[1] Period. In healthy women, this natural process should be relatively simple. I've witnessed women who undergo menopause with few difficulties; in fact, most of them are delighted to finally be done with menstruation. Unfortunately, it's become a cumbersome, symptomatic process for many women due to poor eating habits, stress, lack of exercise and whole body exhaustion. Flip through any women's health

---

1   Estrogen is a messenger of sexual communication at the cellular level; it carries signals between the reproductive organs and supportive glands.

magazine and you'll be bombarded with articles and ads dealing with menopause.

Recommendations for treatment of hot flashes, night sweats and vaginal dryness include everything from herbal remedies to magnetic bracelets. Following are a list of symptoms of menopause as experienced by most women in our society:

Menopause:

> Lowered estrogen levels.

> Extra fat is deposited in the tissues of the body.

> Possible loss of stature (height) due to bone loss.

> Increase in osteoporosis.

> Elevated risk of breast cancer.[2]

> Symptoms may include depression, anxiety, irritability, mood swings and inability to concentrate.

> Physical symptoms include hot flashes, and night sweats.

> Sexual symptoms include decreased libido, vaginal dryness and urinary problems.

The healthy women I see avoiding these menopausal challenges pursue a lifestyle that includes whole foods, no sugar and optimal thyroid function. They also regularly exercise with the resistance of free weights, machines or bands and receive spinal corrective care. I can't say it enough: **It is possible to walk through menopause and bypass the potential physical and emotional symptoms that plague most of the female population!** Of course, this requires a proactive mindset and the determined goal of good health.

---

2   The risk of breast cancer, from my clinically-based experience, I found increases in patients with elevated estrogen, low iodine levels and compromised liver function.

For years, the focus has been on menopause and how decreased hormone function affects women, but the medical community is just starting to consider that hormonal changes occur in men as well. There is little clinical investigation into the role of hormones in men's health, but the magazines at the grocery store checkout are a clue to the state of hormonal health in our society. Erectile dysfunction has never been so prominent! The days of quiet whispering are over; now ads for pills, creams and pumps scream from the covers of magazines to every blushing consumer.

Have you ever paused to consider if these two issues might be related? Could there actually be a phenomenon called "male menopause?" Science increasingly proves it's true and has named it "Andropause."

Andropause:	Menopause:
Testosterone reduced	Estrogen reduced
Body fat increase	Body fat increase
Biological status decrease	Biological status decrease
Osteoporosis increase	Osteoporosis increase
Cardiovascular dx increase	Cardiovascular dx increase
Prostate cancer increase	Breast Cancer increase

Andropause is a relatively new concept. While male sex hormones may experience a slight decline with age, men were designed to perform sexually and father children indefinitely. You might recall that in the Old Testament, Abraham and Sarah were well past child-bearing age when Isaac was conceived and born. (Abraham was one hundred and Sarah was ninety!) Once again, unhealthy lifestyles complicate the normal decline of hormones during aging, bringing about a whole host of accompanying symptoms.

Andropause:

> Defined as a loss of androgen dominance in men.

> Caused by functional imbalances in the male hormone pathway wherein free testosterone declines 1-2 percent yearly.

> Testosterone is made from cholesterol and plays an important role in supporting the thyroid and healthy triglycerides. Cholesterol-lowering statin drugs are shown to reduce testosterone.

> Symptoms may include: mood swings, depression, and pessimism.

> Physical symptoms include muscle weakness, insulin resistance, hypertension, mid-body fat gain, blood sugar issues, osteoporosis and thin, dry skin.

> Sexual symptoms include decreased libido, erectile dysfunction and prostate/urinary problems.

Androgen is the generic term for any natural or synthetic compound that stimulates or controls the development and maintenance of masculine characteristics by binding to androgen receptors. This includes the activity of the accessory male sex organs (the testes, epididymis and seminal vesicles) and development of male secondary sex characteristics such as facial hair, deepening of the voice, etc. Androgens were first discovered in 1936. They are the original anabolic steroids that have been used by body builders and athletes and are the precursor of female sex hormones, called estrogen. The primary and most well-known androgen is testosterone, which is produced in both sexes.

Testosterone is secreted primarily in the testes of males and the ovaries of females, although small amounts are secreted by the adrenal glands. In both men and women, it plays a key role in libido, energy levels, immunity and protection against osteoporosis.

On average, an adult male produces twenty to thirty times the amount of testosterone that an adult woman does.

If menopause is supposed to be such an easy transition and andropause shouldn't even occur, why are patients dragging themselves into my office with many of the symptoms mentioned above? To be blunt, it's because too many people aren't serious about investing in their health. We plan for retirement, we plan for vacation, we plan for our children's college funds, but somehow the planning it takes to maintain a healthy body falls to the wayside. Think of your body as a bank account. You can put in deposits and create a base of "health wealth," or you can continually make withdrawals until you're finally forced to declare bankruptcy.

When men and women come into my office experiencing symptomatic menopause and andropause, I can almost always pinpoint two basic causes: adrenal gland and thyroid burnout and/or decreased liver function. The adrenal glands are designed to be your steroid hormone backup and your thyroid keeps energy levels high. You can read about these challenges in the Adrenal Gland and Thyroid (Turning Up the Heat) Chapters. In the remainder of this chapter, we'll focus on the major culprits in menopause and andropause challenges.

STRESS

When stress levels are constantly high, they lead to impaired adrenal function. The nutrients for routine cellular function are being used to make cortisone to handle the stress, leaving very little left over to make testosterone and estrogen. Cholesterol production is also diverted to make ever-increasing amounts of cortisone instead of being used for sex-based steroid hormones. The result…symptomatic menopause and andropause.

These patients very often fit the same mold. Their work and personal commitments are extremely demanding, occasionally to the point of physical collapse. The women have reached a point of hormonal exhaustion anywhere between forty and fifty years old, sometimes even earlier. These ladies are raising children, some even grandchildren, caring for the household, working and contributing to the family finances and possibly caring for one or more elderly parents. The men don't have it any easier; they feel trapped by family finances into working extremely long hours at jobs that may include shift changes, business travel and demanding clients. On top of all the responsibilities, both men and women are juggling marriage, child rearing, friendships and commitments to church and community organizations. It's no wonder they're exhausted and taking antidepressants! Add to this confusion the challenges of mixed and blended households and you can understand why patients come staggering into my office looking for help.

A word about financial responsibility is warranted here. Your earning power will never satisfy your yearning desire. That is, no matter how much money you bring in, there will always be one more toy that you'd like to own. I know there are fixed expenses and important investments, but you should do everything you can to minimize your consumption of, and desire for, material possessions. Each new thing you purchase translates into a certain number of hours worked to pay for it.

ALCOHOL AND DRUG USE, PRESCRIPTION MEDICATION

Compounding the stress of daily life is the excessive use of alcohol along with prescription and recreational drugs. Alcohol puts added strain on liver function. Escaping the pressures of life by consuming alcohol and drugs is a slippery slope that can lead to addiction. Over fifty percent of insured Americans are on at least one prescription medication, with many more regularly taking multiple prescriptions each day. These medications treat the symptom while ignoring the cause and come with their own set of side effects. Make the first solution you reach for a natural one.

POOR NUTRITION LEADING TO STRESS ON THE LIVER

Today's typical diet is filled with sugar. The negative effects of sugar are actually more powerful than the positive attributes of wholesome food and quality supplements. You should commit to minimizing your consumption of sugar and sugar substitutes. Processed foods have been stripped of nutrients that are absolutely essential for good health, yet they've become a staple of our diets. We're also consuming higher and higher levels of toxic chemicals which stress the liver. If changes aren't made, both men and women will suffer from the resulting loss of sexual desire and ability to perform as well as general poor health. Your diet should be full of whole foods that provide the nutrients your body needs to maintain good health, and you should be able to pass through menopause unscathed. I suggest you look through The Page Fundamental Diet Plan Appendix 3 for healthy meal ideas.

INSUFFICIENT IODINE

A leading culprit in symptomatic menopause and andropause is insufficient iodine. A quality source of sea minerals is an excellent adjunct to your daily food intake; Celtic Sea Salt® would be an example of a mineral that can be applied liberally to your meals. Kelp and sea vegetables are also a fine source of iodine, and you should avoid hot tubs and pools with bromine and chlorine which are antagonistic to iodine. These supplements will be beneficial if you suffer from dry eyes and chronic sinus challenges. My experience has shown that iodine also decreases PSA readings in men who experience prostate challenges.

INSUFFICIENT ZINC

A zinc deficiency can also be responsible for symptomatic menopause and andropause. I generally see a diminished sense of taste and smell in patients lacking zinc. Sugar, stress, and consuming wheat and soy products all deplete zinc. Memory loss, slow healing, white spots on the nails and impaired insulin function can be precipitated by a zinc deficiency. Zinc is a critical ingredient in prostate function in men.

ESTROGEN SATURATION

An overabundance of estrogen (in both men and women) can in many cases create symptomatic hormonal challenges. You should check your abdomen, arms and legs for small, raised, cherry-colored bumps called "cherry hemangiomas."[3] An abundance of these bumps is a sign of possible estrogen saturation. In men, this translates into prostrate issues and altered libido. You can read about more ways to combat estrogen saturation in the Hormone and Liver Chapters.

Menopause doesn't have to be a dreaded and horrific experience, and aging men shouldn't be assigned to decreased libido and erectile challenges. All of these "pause" symptoms can be avoided by making daily investments into your health bank account. The dividends of maintaining "health wealth" include a great sex life well into old age in addition to the blessing of good health and wonderful golden years.

JUST TELL ME WHAT TO DO

❏ If you're going through menopause, browse the list of symptoms to determine which you are experiencing.

❏ Gentlemen, are you experiencing any of the symptoms of andropause?

❏ Sit down with your calendar and identify activities that can be removed to minimize stress.

❏ Limit or eliminate alcohol consumption and discontinue illegal drug use. Consult with a natural health care professional about natural ways to treat high blood pressure, cholesterol, etc. without the use of

---

3   You can read about this in more detail in the Liver Chapter.

prescription drugs. Don't stop taking these medications without the approval of your doctor.

❑ Eliminate sugar, sugar substitutes and processed foods from your diet. Instead, eat a diet rich in whole foods and organic meats. Consume three to five ounces of protein with each meal. Consult The Page Fundamental Diet Plan Appendix 3 for meal ideas.

❑ For optimal hormonal production, take one tablespoon of flax oil per one hundred pounds of body weight.

❑ Iodine supplementation is critical for long term health. I encourage my patients to take up to twelve milligrams of an iodine/iodide combination daily. You should have either a urine iodine loading test or a urine iodine level assessment to determine iodine levels in your system.

❑ Read the Hormone and Liver Chapters for ways to avoid estrogen saturation.

❑ Supplement with an herbal phytoestrogen and/or a wheat germ capsule.

❑ Tribulus is an herb that will help increase the production of testosterone in men.

❑ Saliva hormone testing is an excellent assessment to evaluate your hormone levels. Available upon request to clients of Dr. DeMaria.

❑ Exercise a minimum of thirty minutes daily. Incorporate aerobic and muscle strength training.

16
Fantasy Land

The Garden of Eden was a literal fantasy land; Adam and Eve enjoyed unity not only with each other but with the Lord. God had created them for each other and placed the couple in a beautiful, unblemished environment to live, love and laugh together.

Satan's strategy for destroying this paradise was to undermine their unity. He deceived Eve into believing she could and should make a decision independently of her husband. As Eve touched the forbidden fruit she died spiritually and lost the glory of God's anointing. For those few moments before Adam took the fruit and they both fell, husband and wife were unequally yoked.[1] What happened next is hidden between the lines of the bible text. Adam could visibly see the result of rebellion as God's glory faded from Eve's countenance. Despite this, Adam still chose to join her in rebellion and took the fruit she offered him. This illustrates just one reason our marriages are so important: it's not just about us! Division or the effects of sin do affect all dimensions of life. Eve wasn't thinking about this when she partook, and neither do we. The anointing they lost

---

1   For a great visual representation of what happened during The Fall, I highly recommend seeing *In the Beginning* at Sight and Sound Theatres.

changed everything for them, and in turn for the rest of humanity.

Satan is at work in much the same way today; he uses the tool of deception and plays with our emotions. He offers a new version of "Fantasy Land" that can be ours if we'll reach for that luscious, forbidden fruit. Don't be deceived — all the demonic forces of hell are bent on destroying the creative power of strong, godly marriages! Some of Satan's most effective tools are the media, songs, advertisements, radio, TV, magazines and movies.[2]

Imagine that two couples go see a romantic comedy and the plot includes a loving husband who sets up romantic situations for his wife to enjoy. A couple who are united in purpose and passion might really enjoy the movie and their time together. Their love for each other is enhanced, leading to a peaceful evening filled with intimate conversation and sexual intimacy. Conversely, a couple experiencing division will be perfect targets for Satan's crafty plans. He might plant seeds of discontentment in the wife's heart. ("My husband would never plan a romantic evening like that for me.") The husband may be attacked with negative emotions as well. ("She's never happy with anything I do anyway, so why should I keep on trying?") While one couple goes home to a peaceful evening filled with sexual intimacy, the other couple's romantic plans are thwarted by perceptions which may or may not even be truthful. A marriage that is consistently marked by division easily plays right into Satan's hands.

Satan loves to deceive us and use our emotions in his attack. If he can take our eyes off the blessings of our marriage for one

---

2   It's interesting to note that scripture calls Satan "The Prince of the Power of the Air" (Eph 2:2). Most of these tools are relayed by sound waves and light waves.

second and offer a *new* Fantasy Land, many will reach for the fruit. And the enticement of the world is great: revealing outfits, sexual escapades, articles on the why, what and how to do it, intimate apparel and 900 numbers are all calling for our attention. Satan convinces us that it's more pleasurable to get a quick sexual fix outside our marriage bed than appreciate what we have within it. Those who fall for the bait lose the immeasurable gift of years of marital fulfillment.

Isn't it funny that the hit shows of today are called "reality" shows, even though television and movies don't portray real life? Finding something decent to watch is almost impossible, especially during the evening sitcoms. They're all based on some sort of sexual function (or dysfunction) and most don't even mention marriage.

In the early years of television, one way for my mom and me to get away from household chores was to escape into soap operas. We quickly got hooked. It was amazing how easily they sucked me in; I felt my own life was unfolding in the storylines. TV producers aren't naive, and they realize that it's possible to capitalize on every person's desire to be loved. (This is a healthy desire that's God-given, by the way.) Watching these shows in my young married life made me an emotional wreck. My marriage didn't have the fun and intensity of the shows and so I slowly began pushing Bob aside and finding comfort and passion in an imaginary Fantasy Land. In hindsight I can recognize Satan's ploy, the same one he used on Eve. "What you have isn't good enough. I can offer you something far better." Like Eve, I made a selfish, independent decision and traded something of true value for a lie. This lie could have totally destroyed my life, but the Holy Spirit's conviction led me to repent, and I completely surrendered the soap opera Fantasy Land to Him. He brought restoration and fulfillment to my life and has used this experience to allow me to minister and preach the truth to others.

It's a sad fact that many people, Christians included, are falling into this trap. The Fantasy Land that Satan offers is everywhere you turn. The choice to believe the lie, to reach out and grasp that fruit, can have lifelong implications. It will also keep you wanting more, because fantasy is a thirst that is never quenched.

So what's the answer to this scheme of Satan? Colossians 3:2 says, "Set your minds and keep them set on what is above (the higher things), not on the things that are on the earth." This isn't simply referring to heaven but also to God's design and plan for your life. We are to focus on *God's* way of doing things. The most obvious and practical method of learning His ways is by spending time reading and studying scripture; in fact, the remainder of Colossians 3 is full of foundational teaching on loving others, so it's a great place to start! The Holy Spirit will faithfully lead you as you approach Him with a humble heart and a willingness to learn how to better love your spouse.

One very practical way to build unity in your marriage and avoid the devil's bait is to consider the words you speak to your mate. Your words flow from the abundance of your heart and reveal much about who you are.[3] In Mark 4:14, Jesus told his disciples to sow the Word. The seed in the Kingdom of God is the Word, and the seeds of your life are your words. That means everything in your life right now is directly related to the words you have spoken. Are you satisfied with the relationship you have with your spouse? One kind word can relieve anxiety and depression. Are you speaking kind words? Proverbs 12:25 states, "Anxiety in the heart of man causes depression. But a good word makes it glad." Sounds like an excellent word to me and a great place to start!

---

3   Luke 6:45

Another way to stop Satan from destroying your marriage with a Fantasy Land is to consider your sexual relationship. Husbands, if you've transferred your passion for your wife to the golf course, fishing boat or bowling alley, your wife is a prime target for Satan. He's probably constructing a customized Fantasy Land attack that will include a man who is attentive to her needs. Ladies, if you're not engaging in a regular sexual relationship with your husband, he's more than likely traipsing off to his own Fantasy Land because you're unavailable. Ask God how you can better serve your spouse in the area of sexual intimacy to extinguish Satan's attacks.

Avoid becoming one of the sad couples who escape to a Fantasy Land and wake up one day to find they've lost everything valuable in the meantime. Ask God to give you contentment in your marriage right now, no matter what state it's in, and don't let a fantasy kill your dream. Every day can be a walk in the garden.

JUST TELL ME WHAT TO DO

- ❑ Commit to focus your thoughts on reality and not a fantasy.
- ❑ Guard your mind. Turn off the TV and be cautious about the movies you watch.
- ❑ Confess any ways you've bought into and embraced Satan's Fantasy Land. Make a plan to break free from any habits you may have established.
- ❑ Read Colossians Chapter 3 with your mate.

17
Stay In the Lines!!
Creating a Faithful Marriage Relationship

I t's become a common occurrence in our society for a
husband or wife to have numerous affairs, desert their
spouse and children and move in with another willing
partner. They leave behind a train wreck of shattered hopes,
dreams and lives in their wake, oblivious to anyone's needs but
their own. Divorce after divorce results in the legacy of a
generational curse that impacts lineages far beyond the ones
directly involved. Battles over custody, possessions and
visitation turn the whole experience into a long and drawn out
war instead of the simple "solution" that many couples claim
they are seeking.

As resilient as we claim they are, children aren't unaffected
by even the neatest of separations and divorces. Willing or not,
they are often dragged away from parents, grandparents,
schoolmates, and familiar neighborhoods. The separation
anxiety alone can generate lifelong emotional scars. I see the
results in my practice often. It's very challenging as a natural
health care provider to restore physical ailments that have an
emotional source from years of unforgiveness and bitterness.

I've treated patients who have genuine physical, emotional
and social impairments due to infidelity, divorce and/or
separation. Many of them have shared the confusion over being

in a nurturing environment one day and suddenly being thrust into stressful living arrangements the next. Some were left with one parent, others felt torn as they were shuttled between two homes, and many were forced to live with a parent's new lover who was a complete stranger to them. All of this heartache was caused by the emotional, endorphin-charged high of a parent's inappropriate sexual encounter. Affairs that are consummated in a matter of minutes have a ripple effect that impacts children and families for years to come, and the natural order of things can never be restored as it once was.

The consequences of a moment of passionate infidelity reach far beyond just the family involved. Remarkably, churches, communities, businesses and even governments can be negatively impacted by extramarital affairs.

I've had many patients come to the office suffering from recurrent, painful symptoms caused by sexually transmitted diseases they contracted from an unfaithful spouse. I've treated wives with herpes and pelvic inflammatory disease struggling with the physical pain of these conditions in addition to the immense emotional hurt of learning their spouse was with another partner. The word of God says that when a person commits a sexual sin, they sin against their own body. The consequences reach far beyond as their selfish pursuits satisfying a moment of passion create heartache and agony for an innocent spouse. Please seriously consider the long-term ramifications if you are contemplating a rendezvous with someone other than your husband or wife. Sexual intimacy should be reserved for your mate alone. Deb and I are amazed by how some married people carry on with others' spouses. We urge you to never let your guard down and be swayed by temptation!

Scripture is clear about immorality in 1 Corinthians 6:12-18 (NIV):

"Everything is permissible for me"—but not everything is beneficial. "Everything is permissible for me"—but I will not be mastered by anything. "Food for the stomach and the stomach for food"—but God will destroy them both. The body is not meant for sexual immorality, but for the Lord, and the Lord for the body. By his power God raised the Lord from the dead and he will raise us also. Do you not know that your bodies are members of Christ himself? Shall I then take the members of Christ and unite them with a prostitute? Never! Do you not know that he who unites himself with a prostitute is one with her in body? For it is said, "The two will become one flesh." But he who unites himself with the Lord is one with him in spirit. Flee from sexual immorality. **All other sins a man commits are outside his body, but he who sins sexually sins against his own body.** *Do you not know that your body is a temple of the Holy Spirit, who is in you, whom you have received from God? You are not your own; you were bought at a price. Therefore honor God with your body.*

How do you protect your marriage? I suggest you start by carefully reading The Hunt Chapter and commit to pursuing your spouse minute by minute. Your marriage isn't a game and should be treated as the precious gift from God that it truly is. Let's consider together what Proverbs 5 has to say about protecting your marriage and staying far from unfaithfulness. You'll find my comments after each verse. (This chapter speaks of a man being warned not to fall into sexual sin with a woman, but it can be applied to both sexes.)

Proverbs 5: Warning against unfaithfulness

1. *My son, pay attention to my wisdom, listen well to my words of insight,*
   Listen to your conscience; don't let it be hardened or silenced due to indifference or disobedience.

2. *that you may maintain discretion and your lips may preserve knowledge.*

Speak prudently and discreetly with others of the opposite sex. (No discussions about sexuality or other inappropriate topics.) Don't be flirtatious in your conversation with another's spouse or an unmarried person.

3. *For the lips of an adulteress drip honey, and her speech is smoother than oil;*
   Don't be flattered and swayed by compliments or the attention of anyone other than your spouse. Don't kiss anyone but your mate, either affectionately or passionately.

4. *But in the end she is bitter as gall, sharp as a double-edged sword.*
   Sexual affairs cut to the heart of all those involved.

5. *Her feet go down to death; her steps lead straight to the grave.*
   Fornication ensnares you and may eventually lead to spiritual death.

6. *She gives no thought to the way of life, her paths are crooked, but she knows it not.*
   Those who welcome illicit affairs either don't care about or are unaware of the consequences of their actions. They are commonly motivated by lust rather than wisdom or godliness.

7. *Now then, my sons listen to me; do not turn aside from what I say.*
   Don't reject or disdain wisdom or godly counsel.

8. *Keep to a path far from her; do not go near the door of her house;*
   Don't give in to temptation in any way, no matter how small or seemingly innocent. Always keep your distance from potentially tempting situations or people.

9. *lest you give your best strength to others and your years to one who is cruel,*
   Anyone who will intentionally become sexually involved with a married man or woman is partnering with evil and cruelty, no matter how "wonderful" they may seem at the time.

10. *lest strangers feast on your wealth and your toil enrich another man's house.*

    Your unfaithfulness can result in divorce and the loss of your assets to another.

11. *At the end of your life you will groan, when your flesh and body are spent.*

    Sinful choices often result in physical consequences, including painful and embarrassing sexually transmitted diseases.

12. *You will say, "How I hated discipline! How my heart spurned correction..."*

    You will eventually regret your ungodly decision but it will be too late to change what you've done.

13. *"....I would not obey my teachers or listen to my instructors."*

    Don't think you're above sexual sin. Don't let your guard down because you believe you're immune to it.

14. *"I have come to the brink of utter ruin in the midst of the whole assembly."*

    If nothing else will motivate you to avoid an affair, consider what others will think of you when they discover your actions.

15. *Drink water from your own cistern, running water from your own well.*

    You do not want to forsake the time spent and energy to establish your own source of refreshment from the well of passion you once had. Stay at home and do not go to another's reservoir. There are consequences to choices.

16. *Should your springs overflow in the streets, your streams of water in the public squares?*

    Stay home, you do need your private personal marital life be a spectacle to all. Do not leave the nest.

17. *Let them be yours alone, never to be shared with strangers.*

   Your sexual needs should be met solely within your marriage by your spouse. A husband and wife have the privilege of being joint owners of their sexual relationship, a precious gift they're not required to share with anyone else! Why should another person get to enjoy the sexual favor of a married partner when their spouse has invested so much love, time and energy in their relationship over the years? Jealously guard your marriage relationship!

18. *May your fountain be blessed, and may you rejoice in the wife of your youth.*

   Enjoy the creativity that results from a satisfied marriage (see the Created to Create Chapter) and continually recall what made you fall in love with your spouse and your early passion for each other.

19. *A loving doe, a graceful deer — may her breasts satisfy you always, may you ever be captivated by her love.*

   Intentionally focus on your spouse's strengths. Delight in their femininity or masculinity. Find physical satisfaction in their body and emotional satisfaction in their love.

20. *Why be captivated, my son, by an adulteress? Why embrace the bosom of another man's wife?*

   When you experience the blessings of a committed marriage, what good reason is there to stray from it? You have all you need at home! You should never have any kind of sexual contact with anyone other than your spouse.

21. *For a man's ways are in full view of the LORD, and he examines all his paths.*

   God clearly sees all of your thoughts, motives and actions. Avoid all of the spiritual, physical and emotional consequences that result from an affair. The guilt and condemnation that follow sexual sin will wreak havoc on your mind and body.

22. *The evil deeds of a wicked man ensnare him; the cords of his sin hold him fast.*

   It's been said that sin will blind you, bind you and grind you. Don't become a prisoner to your desires for someone other than your mate. If you're currently in an ungodly relationship, confess it to God, turn away from it and seek healing in your marriage.

23. *He will die for lack of discipline, led astray by his own great folly.*

   A lack of discipline results in foolish choices that may lead to spiritual and even physical death. A disciplined life leads to freedom.

I hope these verses have showed you just how dangerous sexual sin can be. Writer Arnold Glasow said, "Temptation usually comes in through a door that has been deliberately left open." Most people who have affairs will admit that they didn't suddenly find themselves in bed with their lover. Inappropriate relationships start when we entertain *inappropriate thoughts* that should be rejected from the first moment they enter our minds.[1] That's why it's so important that you and your spouse agree on some very basic ways to protect your marriage *before* either of you are at a point of no return:

> ➤ Pray together every day. This provides a hedge of protection around your marriage and family. It also keeps your hearts in tune as you daily take victories and struggles before God's throne together.

---

1 2Corinthians 10:5 says, "We are destroying speculations and **every** lofty thing raised up against the knowledge of God, and we are taking **every thought captive** to the obedience of Christ."

➤ Find some kind of devotional or an uplifting, faith-filled book and read a page or two together each day.

➤ Never flirt with the opposite sex, no matter how innocent it appears.

➤ Alcohol and drugs lower your inhibitions and often result in licentious behavior that will cause regret later. Agree to avoid these activities without your spouse present or at the least discuss when they should be limited. (Of course, you shouldn't use recreational drugs for a variety of reasons, including this one.)

➤ Don't watch television shows and movies that promote sexual encounters between unmarried characters. I know this rules out just about every primetime show and every movie with a rating over 'G.' If your marriage is a priority you'll be willing to pay the price that faithfulness costs. Your mind is easily influenced and you don't want to leave any doors open that might allow unhealthy fantasies to breed in your heart.

➤ Find ways to build up your spouse so they don't feel needy and unloved. Husbands and wives who don't feel valued are easy prey for others who will flatter them and fill the gaping holes in their hearts. Speak encouraging words, serve them with humility and make your spouse never even want to consider being with anyone else!

➤ If your marriage is struggling, don't share your frustrations with someone of the opposite sex. Instead, seek out a qualified Christian counselor or mentor who can help you find godly solutions.

➤ I strongly advise against working out at co-ed gym facilities *unless you attend with your spouse*. We can all benefit from the accountability that having our partner around brings while surrounded by temptation. Instead of creating a fantasy about the person on the treadmill in front of you, watch your spouse work out and fantasize about your plans when you arrive back home!

➢ Agree that you'll not look at *any kind* of pornographic materials either together or separately. This includes still pictures, videos and even lingerie catalogs. All of these have the potential to create feelings of discontentment with your spouse and lure you away from your marriage. I've seen this happen time and time again to both men and women.

➢ If you travel for business or have business meetings that involve the opposite sex, I encourage you to have a prayer covering and an accountability partner. It's very easy for feelings to develop between business associates.

Your marriage is a precious gift from God. At the end of your life, you'll be blessed to look back at a long, satisfying, wonderful relationship if you make the effort now to protect your marriage and remain faithful partners. God, who is the best example of faithfulness, has promised to give us the strength we need to be loyal partners. Ask Him to help you remain true to the one you made your vows to!

JUST TELL ME WHAT TO DO

❑ Have you been impacted by infidelity, separation or divorce? Discuss what ways you've been affected.

❑ Have you committed sexual sins in the past? If so, confess them to God. (You should talk with a qualified counselor before sharing past indiscretions with your spouse. Sometimes divulging every detail is more harmful than helpful.)

❑ Read Proverbs 5 together and ask God to help you humbly accept His counsel.

❑ Read through the list of ways to protect your marriage. Agree to start putting a few of the ideas into place in your relationship.

18

Planning for Your Wedding...Night!

After over 50 years of observing people from all walks of life, I've come to the conclusion that most people take more time to plan a party than to plan their life. The party they usually spend the most time planning is their wedding. The bride especially goes to great detail arranging everything — from the dresses and tuxedoes to the flowers, favors, and centerpieces. It's even becoming common for couples to hire a wedding planner to ensure that the whole day runs smoothly.

The significance of a wedding deserves such attention and the months preceding the ceremony are an exciting time for both bride and groom as they anticipate becoming one. Commonly lost in the hustle and bustle, however, is preparation for the sexual component of marriage. There seems to be a mindset that because sex is natural, it will just take care of itself on the wedding night and the many nights that follow. Nothing could be further from the truth!

When we were getting married, no one sat us down either individually or as a couple and talked to us about sex. There may have been a few people who wondered if we were ready for this most intimate experience, but no one was brave enough to broach the subject. We *did* get a lot of jokes, teasing and sly winks, but what we most needed was just one mature, sensitive adult who was willing to talk to us lovingly and honestly about our sex life as a couple. If you haven't had this helpful conversation, would you allow me the privilege of being that person who talks candidly with you and gently prepares you for a wonderful start to your sexual life together? I also highly recommend that you find an experienced couple who can help answer any questions you might have in response to this chapter. Seek out a husband and wife who obviously have strong feelings of love and respect for each other. If they commonly touch each other, smile at each other, and seem pleased to be together, they're the couple for you! Of course, you should also feel comfortable with them and trust that everything you share will be held in highest confidence. Having other people present while you discuss intimate issues will help you avoid falling into sexual temptation while you talk about being intimate. And I guarantee that this time spent preparing will leave you satisfied on your wedding night and ready for many more passionate sexual encounters!

A healthy marriage requires two people who are physically drawn together by an indescribable sexual chemistry. Of course, there are other equally important similarities that should attract you to each other, but we are focusing on the sexual component of your relationship. This chemistry works like a magnet between a husband and wife. It's more than simply wanting to be with someone all the time — you actually desire to consume them and be consumed yourself. It's very healthy to have strong sexual desire for your fiancé, even though that desire may make sexual purity a difficult challenge. But the feeling that you can't keep your hands off each other is a good one to take into the marriage bed; it exhibits your God-given attraction to the person He has chosen for you. In fact, if you *don't* feel a strong sexual attraction to the person you're planning to marry, I'd caution you to carefully consider whether you should make the trip down the aisle. It's certainly possible to have a best friend that you aren't sexually attracted to, but that friendship doesn't necessarily mean you should jump to the "I Do's," and you may be better off remaining friends. We're most definitely best friends today, but most of that friendship developed in the years *after* our marriage as we walked together through struggles, challenges, trials and victories. I have to admit that it was in large part our sexual attraction (coupled with common goals and compatibility) that drove us toward the altar. There's no shame in admitting such a fact, as the Apostle Paul himself stated in 1 Corinthians 7:9 that it is "….better to marry than to burn with passion."

Following are a list of topics that you should discuss together in the presence of your mentor couple. After you each have a chance to respond, ask your mentors if they would like to add any comments or advice before moving on to the next topic.

SEX VERSUS ROMANCE

Sex and romance sound like the same thing, but they're most definitely not. It's entirely possible to have sex without feeling romantic and to be romantic without having sex. From our experience and the experience of thousands of married couples, the best intimate moments occur when both sex and romance are present simultaneously. Most dating couples have a solid mix of both romance and sexual attraction during their courtship, so your relationship is likely well-balanced between the two. Later in marriage, most men put higher emphasis on sex while their wives generally desire romance. But even so, combining the two on your wedding night is a sure way to leave smiles on both of your faces. Take turns defining both "sex" and "romance" and talk about ways to incorporate both on that first intimate evening.

YOUR SEXUAL UPBRINGING

How much do you know about sex, where did you learn it from, and how has it shaped your attitude? If you come from a healthy, loving family, you probably learned much about sexuality from your parents. This is a wonderful blessing that will reap huge dividends in your own marriage! If, on the other hand, you picked up your sex education from whispered conversations in the locker room or from watching soap operas, much of what you learned is bound to be only half truths. As crazy as it sounds, it might benefit you to visit your local library and pick up some books that have been written to teach young people about sexuality. At the least, you should understand the basic sexual anatomy of both genders and what's located where. After you've done this, schedule to meet with your mentor couple and split into two groups (ladies and men) for a candid conversation about the ins and outs of intercourse. (Yes, that pun was intentional!)

How did your sexual education mold your attitudes toward intimacy? Are you anticipating your wedding night? Fearful of it? Dreading it? Anticipation is the attitude you want to have approaching this wonderfully intimate act. If you're fearful, lots of honest discussion with your mentor couple will do much to appease your concerns. If you're dreading it due to negative feelings about sexuality or any kind of inappropriate touching or abuse, we strongly suggest you meet with a Christian counselor or pastor. Take whatever steps are necessary to approach your wedding night with joyful anticipation; it will become a precious memory that lasts your whole marriage and your goal should be to make it as wonderful as God intended.

PREPARING FOR THE WEDDING NIGHT

There are some practical decisions that can and should be made to ensure that you have a great first experience. If you plan on using birth control, decide what type, purchase it and learn how it works. Nothing spoils the mood faster than worrying that you might get pregnant sooner that you've hoped or planned.

Decide where and when you'll spend that first night. If you're having an evening wedding, it might make more sense to stay one night in a local hotel before jumping on a plane for your honeymoon. In fact, we've heard of couples who actually *put off* their first act of intercourse until the following morning because they were exhausted from the day's events!

Both of you might plan some romantic gestures such as candles and lingerie. Many couples find this is a nice way to anticipate the moment and surprise their new spouse, but looking back it's usually not necessary for an exciting sexual experience. Plainly put, you'll probably be so turned on by the mere sight of each other naked that you won't even remember to light the candles or put on the lingerie! It's something you'll look back on and laugh about years later when romance becomes a much more necessary ingredient in mutually satisfying encounters.

FOR THE GROOM

Congratulations, gentlemen, on sweeping your bride off her feet! God has now given you the privilege of pleasing and protecting your new wife. Many men forego this responsibility as they quickly jump to meet their own sexual needs without thinking of their spouse. You, on the other hand, have already shown consideration for her simply by reading this book.

Probably the biggest challenge you'll face on your first night together will be holding back your rush of sexual excitement and slowing down enough to make the night pleasurable for the both of you. I can't overstate the importance of creating a wonderful memory for your wife. She will remember every detail of this night; even the things you think are insignificant. Years from now, she'll be able to tell you the color of the wallpaper, what kind of underwear you were wearing, and more importantly, how she felt about the sexual experience. Women tend to be much more delicate than men. This means you should strive to be sensitive to her needs and feelings and your touches should always be tender. Proverbs 5:18-19 says, "May your fountain be blessed, and may you rejoice in the wife of your youth. A loving doe, a graceful deer — may her breasts satisfy you always, may you ever be captivated by her love."

Your blushing bride will probably be a bit nervous and may also be shy about her nakedness. Respond with compassion by dimming the lights and assuring her of your love. Instead of jumping right to the main event, kiss her, stroke her hair, run your hands over her back. Tell her how much you've longed to be with her. Women are very responsive to verbal communication, so don't be silent or it will only add to her nervousness. She'll replay the words you speak on this night for years to come.

You should always be listening for your wife's responses to your touches; this is the best way to learn what she does and doesn't enjoy. Anytime she pulls back from a touch should signal you to try something different. This might be as subtle as her sudden silence or as obvious as her hands guiding you away from a certain area of her body. But by all means, enjoy exploring her whole body with your hands and mouth and let her cues guide you! Many couples incorrectly view sex as a one dish meal consisting of penis inside vagina. On the contrary, your bodies are a buffet of wonderful foods that were made to be touched and tasted in any manner that is pleasurable for both of you!

Your wife will probably be touching your body as well during this time. It's a temptation for many men to become lost in their own pleasure, which may lead to premature ejaculation and an incredibly quick sexual experience. Try to keep the whole lovemaking session mutually pleasurable. If you sense an impending ejaculation, it's okay to put your hand on hers and ask her to stop stimulating your penis for a while. To avoid offending her, you should quietly whisper something like, "You're turning me on so much but I want to make this last. Why don't you let me focus on touching you for awhile so that we can both be satisfied." (Some of you are thinking, "Do I really have to write all of these comments on index cards and tape them on the wall?!" Of course you don't have to memorize these exact words; I'm just trying to give you some ideas of gentle ways to communicate to your wife that will not offend her delicate emotions.)

If you sense your wife doesn't really know what to do with your body, give her subtle hints by guiding her hands to places you'd like to be touched. You might even wrap your hands around hers and show her how quickly or slowly she should stroke. Many women appreciate these clues and will delight in learning how to delight you.

As your foreplay becomes more passionate, you might start to rub your penis against her external genitals. There are two obvious signs that she is ready for penetration. The first is that she will be *asking you* to enter her! Many women feel a very strong longing for penetration and will verbally ask for it or even take matters into their own hands by pulling you inside themselves. The second sign is that she will have vaginal lubrication. You can find this out by gently running your fingers over her external genitalia and/or vaginal entrance. It won't be difficult to determine, as lubricated vaginas are generally very wet and unlubricated vaginas are very dry! If you've been kissing and touching each other for a considerable amount of time and she is still dry, ask her if she'd like you to use some lubricating jelly. You should have some on hand.

After you penetrate your wife, your body will naturally want to thrust quickly in and out of her. Do everything you can to fight this impulse! First of all, she needs you to start very gently, and secondly, you want to avoid ejaculating too quickly. Listen and feel for her cues. It's perfectly okay to slow down or even stop thrusting for a time and regain control by touching her in other ways. In fact, switching from thrusting to kissing to stroking her breasts is incredibly stimulating for most women.

When you sense that ejaculation is imminent, let her know. Many women find this very exciting and will want to share in the experience with you. Communicate how good it feels! It can be disappointing for a woman to discover that, unbeknownst to her, her husband has quietly finished and she was unaware that he was even ejaculating. Let her enjoy your orgasm as much as you do! Then (as discussed below in the Let's Be Real section) get her some tissues, allow her to go to the bathroom if she needs to, and spend lots of time holding each other and basking in the afterglow of your first night together.

FOR THE BRIDE

If you're like most women, you've been dreaming about your wedding and wedding night for most of your life. And now here it is! All of the planning is finished and you're finally free to offer your body to your new husband and give him the most intense pleasure he will ever experience. A huge part of that pleasure for men is the knowledge that *you* are enjoying yourself and that he is able to turn you on. For this reason, I can't stress enough that you *communicate* your pleasure to him. Respond to what feels good by whispers and sighs and by moving your body against his. It will drive him crazy! As your lovemaking becomes more passionate, feel free to explore his whole body with your hands and mouth. If you're unsure what to do or what he would enjoy, ask him! Run your hands over his back and his buttocks, his nipples and his neck. Whisper how much you love him and that his body feels so good next to yours. Eventually your focus will turn to his penis. Gently stroke it with your hands, but be careful to follow his cues. If he asks you to slow down or stops your hands with his, he may be approaching ejaculation and you should temporarily stop and allow him to regain control. If he asks you to touch him in a specific way and it is something that you find appealing, go ahead and please him! If you're unsure of yourself, graciously communicate it to him or ask him if you can talk about it later. "Can I try this instead?" is a gentle way of turning down a request you feel uncomfortable meeting.

Your husband may be unsure about how you would like to be touched, and that's perfectly okay. Direct him with whispers or by simply moving his hands where you'd like to be stroked. He may even be unsure about penetration and worried about hurting you. It's fine for you to guide his penis inside you with your hands. In fact, a wonderful way to facilitate that first experience is for you to straddle him and slowly lower yourself onto his penis. This allows you to guide the rate that he enters you and control the depth of his thrusts. It's also very visually stimulating for him to see your whole body as you make love. Look into his eyes as he enters you and be fully aware that in this moment the two of you are physically becoming one flesh in God's sight.

If you sense the ability to have an orgasm, let him know and guide him in bringing it about. Don't feel pressured to perform, though. If you don't feel an orgasm is possible tonight, quietly let him know that there will be other times and you just want to enjoy having him inside of you. Most women don't require an orgasm to have a satisfying sexual experience; just the intimacy of the act is very fulfilling. Occasionally a woman's clitoris will become somewhat tired from lengthy stimulation and can even become irritated. If this occurs, you should move his hands to a different part of your body and let him know that you'd like to try that at a different time. "I just want to enjoy your orgasm this time," is a wonderful way to communicate your longing for him without offending his ego.

A man's orgasm is a large turn-on for most women, so tell him that you want to know when he ejaculates. Help him understand that you are looking forward to this exhilarating moment and you want to share it with him. His penis will become very hard as he ejaculates and this can be a very pleasurable sensation as he moves it inside of you.

A NOTE ABOUT KISSING

Kissing — especially French kissing — is an intimate part of the sexual act. The dance of lips and tongues is a re-enactment of intercourse in miniature! For this reason, women tend to respond most to gentle kisses. One of the biggest turnoffs for women is a man who roughly thrusts his tongue in and out of their mouth and covers her with his sloppy, wet saliva. This is simply a sign of his desire to thrust something *else* in and out of her, but it tends to get messy and rough! Grooms, you should treat kissing just as you do penetration: slowly, gently, and tenderly. Trust me, if you kiss your wife this way, she will be *begging* for penetration by the time you get there!

LET'S BE REAL

I want to share something about the sexual experience that I can guarantee you have never seen in a movie. After a man ejaculates inside a woman, the semen has to go somewhere, and that place is…back out. (What goes up must come down.) You will want to have some tissues nearby just for this moment. (We have friends who keep a few small hand towels in their night side drawer.) Husbands, it will really bless your wife if you take on the responsibility of getting her some tissues or a towel after you're done making love. She will appreciate having something to catch your semen in as she makes her way to the bathroom. And ladies, it's always a good idea to urinate after sex anyway to avoid the possibility of urinary tract infections, plus it will give the remaining semen a chance to come out into the toilet. I know this isn't a very romantic topic, but couples have been dealing with "overflow" throughout all of history and being prepared will help you avoid the embarrassment of discovering it on your own that first night together. The tissues will also come in handy if you experience premature ejaculation and release semen outside of your wife's vagina. If this happens, don't panic! Remember to set your expectations high for preparation but realistically low for execution. You may not feel this way at the time, but trust me: you will look back and chuckle over your wedding night about a thousand times during the course of your marriage.

While we are talking about the practical side of sex, you should decide on a form of birth control and know how it works. This can be awkward but if you approach the night with grace and an intact sense of humor it won't cause any problems.

Additionally, remember that there's no script to be followed. You might end up making love in the bedroom; you might not be able to wait that long and the kitchen table might seem pretty inviting as you walk in the door! The most important goal is that you enjoy each other's bodies and make this a wonderful experience. If you wake up at midnight feeling frisky, go for Round Two! Your wedding night will be as unique as you are.

SET THE STANDARDS HIGH...AND LOW!

You should have high standards for your wedding night, meaning you should both be prepared and ready to please and be pleased. At the same time, expecting the kind of sexual earthquakes and fireworks you see in movies is going to set you up for disappointment because *those movie scenes tend to be unrealistic.* No, most women do not want to be thrown over the hood of a car and taken in a moment of passion. No, dual orgasms generally don't occur within three minutes. In fact, as good as your wedding night can be, the greatest married sex takes time to learn. Years from now, your wedding night will be a precious memory but probably won't be your greatest intimate moment. Husbands, you should work towards the goal of giving your new wife an orgasm, but neither of you should be disappointed if it doesn't happen. Expecting it can place undue pressure on both of you and will almost guarantee a frustrating intimate time that may leave either of you raw and aching. There will be many more opportunities in your marriage, so if this night is over quickly, remember that the morning will generally bring another erection and the desire for more! Your wedding night is only the start of a wonderful sexual journey for both of you.

THE SECOND TIME AROUND

Not every wedding night will be a first sexual encounter. If the two of you have already had sex together or with someone else (yes, this happens in our imperfect world), you should still make preparations for this to be a special time. Others are preparing for second marriages or have had prior sexual experiences with boyfriends or girlfriends. This is increasingly common today, but we still hope and pray that whatever your past has held, this night will be a wonderful time for both of you. You've entered into a covenant with each other and with God, and the consummation of your marriage seals the deal. It's an act that should be held in high regard regardless of the past.

Many couples who have had sex before their wedding night, whether with each other or in past relationships, have shared a common struggle with us: There's a large temptation to compare the wedding night with previous sexual partners. We encourage you to avoid this at all costs and to focus instead on your feelings of love for your new spouse and what they bring to your relationship. Unconditional love will not judge or rate; it accepts completely without conditions. If you find yourself struggling to love unconditionally, ask God to help you find satisfaction in your spouse. Here is the chance to start fresh. You've had the opportunity to learn from past mistakes, and God is able to redeem all that we offer Him. As an old song said, "He can even make it 'feel like the first time!'"

God created sex to be one of the greatest blessings of marriage and a physical representation of how we become one spiritually in this holy union. He said it is good, and we know that your experience together will confirm this is so! Approach your wedding night with practical preparation, fully anticipating that it will be the wonderful and pleasurable experience God intended.

JUST TELL ME WHAT TO DO

☐ Find a mature, experienced couple who you both trust and respect. Ask if they would consider meeting with you to prepare for your sexual relationship.

☐ Discuss your attitudes about sex. What was modeled in your families? What are your honest expectations for your first night together? Ask your mentor couple if they feel your expectations are realistic or if they may need to be adjusted.

☐ Do you have any specific likes and dislikes that should be communicated before your wedding night? Are there any sexual acts that you feel inhibited about performing? Are there any you are especially looking forward to?

☐ If you plan to use birth control, determine what method, obtain it and understand how it works.

☐ Relax, take your time, and enjoy each other!

19

Talking to Your Kids About Sex

The sexual education of your children goes far beyond the words of a health textbook and shouldn't be outlined or measured by the opinions of teachers, no matter how good their intentions. It also starts long before seventh grade health class and isn't learned in one semester from a book or a teacher. Sex education begins with the sexual climate and attitudes in your own home.

Information about sexuality is "caught" more than "taught." Years before your children begin to understand the dynamics of a sexual relationship, they form attitudes about gender, touch and intimacy. You have the opportunity to assist in building a godly and healthy sexual foundation that will bless your children for a lifetime.

CHILDREN ADOPT THE STANDARDS OF THEIR PARENTS

Regardless of what you say (or don't say), your children are absorbing your values and standards every minute of the day. This includes what you intentionally teach them and what you simply avoid or allow to enter your home, conversations and lifestyle. If Dad keeps pornography in the home office, the children will accept that this is appropriate whether it's ever brought up in conversation or not. If Mom wears suggestive clothing, her teenage daughters may in time choose similar outfits. The same is true for the television programs and movies you watch. Even if they contain questionable material that you wouldn't personally advocate, if you allow them to be viewed in your home, you're sending a silent message to your children that what's happening on the screen is acceptable behavior. Children's hearts and minds are incredibly absorbent. Make it a high priority to guard them and put godly standards in place that will guide their relationships throughout their lifetime.

MODELING APPROPRIATE TOUCHING

It's natural to want to hold and snuggle your babies and toddlers and this intimate touching actually has health benefits for both children and parents. It's also sobering to realize that some children may eventually reach a point where they're uncomfortable being hugged by Mom and Dad. Even if this occurs, parents should continue modeling healthy touching while being sensitive to their son's or daughter's feelings. This continual display of affection will establish a healthy foundation for their own future relationships, eventually leading to healthy sex lives.

The way you tenderly hold your children sends a strong message to them that touching is good, pleasurable and an expression of love. On the contrary, children who are physically abused may relate their negative experience to touching of any form, including future marital sexual encounters. You can see why it's so important in these formative years to make hugging a normal part of your children's day. Other forms of normal and healthy touching include hand holding, play wrestling and kissing. Children should be taught that kissing Mom, Dad and siblings is natural and appropriate, but touching those outside of the family is done in less intimate ways. These subtle differences help children recognize that certain forms of touching are more intimate than others. It will also protect kids as well as the rest of the family from exposure to viruses and germs!

Don't be concerned if your children exhibit differing levels of physical affection. Regardless of their gender, certain boys and girls are more affectionate while others pull back from long embraces. As long as these reactions aren't the result of inappropriate experiences, your children will express what they feel comfortable with in their own unique ways.

MODELING APPROPRIATE INTIMACY

Obviously, the ways we touch our spouse are far more intimate than how we hold our children. It's unfortunate our kids aren't allowed to get a glimpse into those intimate moments as couples. This doesn't mean that you and your spouse should leave the bedroom door unlocked; in fact, I highly recommend that you install a lock on your door if you don't have one there already. Learning that the two of you have sex in theory is much less threatening than walking in on an intimate moment! (It generally takes years for kids to get over the "creepiness" of Mom and Dad having sexual desires for each other.)

Intimate touches between parents that are appropriate for children to see include hugs, kisses, hand holding, gentle "love pats" and snuggling. Children desperately need the security of knowing that their Mom and Dad love each other and their family is stable and intact. Every intimate gesture affirms this truth and brings peace to a child's heart.

When conflicts arise between you and your spouse, make sure your children see you make up. Make it a point to hug in front of the children and verbally remind them, "Mom and Dad might disagree sometimes and even fight, but we still love each other very much." As you embrace each other, younger children especially may run up and join in a "family hug." Their hearts find security in seeing parents who value their relationship and are willing to work hard for their marriage and the family as a whole.

"MY BODY BELONGS TO ME, YOUR BODY BELONGS TO YOU"

One of our friends has used this simple phrase to teach her youngsters about appropriate touching, modesty and stranger issues. Toddlers already believe that everything belongs to them ("Mine!") and this requires no stretch of their imaginations.[1] Start by telling your children at an early age that their bodies belong to them. They will quickly develop a sense of pride and privacy in their beautiful little bodies. Modesty is a simple issue: "If your body belongs to you, should you be showing it to anyone else?[2]" There's no embarrassment in this type of conversation that focuses on the goodness of their bodies instead of suggesting that displaying them is shameful. (After all, you want your grown children to eventually find great pleasure in undressing with their future spouse.) In addition, adults should model modesty and explain to the children that Mom and Dad's bodies belong to Mom and Dad alone as well, and there's no reason for children to watch their parents dressing or undressing. (Of course, there are precious times when children are babies that you may climb in the tub with them, but those bath times should stop long before they gain an awareness of sexuality and private parts.)

Maintaining high standards in what you watch on television and in movie theatres follows the same simple principle. If a woman is scantily clad, discuss who her body belongs to. If that actress's body belongs only to her, you might ask why she would want to share it with the whole world. There's no shame involved and you will avoid sending the message that nakedness is "bad," only that it is private and precious.

Our friend who came up with the "Your body belongs to you" phrase happens to have two daughters. She and her husband started praying for their future husbands as soon as their little girls were born, including these thoughts in bedtime prayers in front of their children. As a result, their daughters have become

---

1   Of course, as adults we understand that their bodies belong to God, but at young ages and for these teaching purposes the phrase is helpful and fitting.
2   Children should be taught that it's all right for a doctor to view their bodies during a physical exam.

very aware that some day they *will* have the opportunity to share their bodies with another person: their husbands. But for the time being, they understand that Mom and Dad are helping to protect their bodies until that time when they are offered as a beautiful gift to the men who win their hearts. Whether you have boys or girls, make sure that at the appropriate age your children understand the purpose for keeping their bodies private and protected: so they can eventually give the precious gift of their virginity to their spouse.

EMBRACING APPROPRIATE GENDER ROLES

Our children are growing up in a society filled with increasingly warped and confused gender roles. They're bombarded with negative statements about both sexes and resentment over the challenges each gender faces. We know that God was intentional in every detail of his creation — including gender — and he called it "good." As your kids participate in co-ed sports teams and activities, they will quickly learn to relate to both sexes while at the same time finding a unique way to express their own femininity and masculinity. And of course, each child will be different as a result of their personality and preferences. You may have a daughter who insists on wearing dresses every day and another who wrinkles her nose at the thought of putting on anything other than blue jeans. Some boys live for sports while others prefer concentrating on their studies or artistic hobbies. Regardless of their preferences in these areas, the goal is for each child to embrace their gender and avoid any kind of resentment or confusion over how they were created.

SEXUAL ANATOMY AND EDUCATION

As you teach your kids about their bodies in those very early years, I encourage you to use correct anatomy terms. "Wee wee" may sound cute now, but at some point your child may need to express a need to another adult who might have no idea what "wee wee" means. Using proper names also demystifies the sexual organs when the time comes for the birds and bees talk.

And speaking of this impending conversation, it's been my experience that it won't happen all at once but will be slowly revealed over a matter of months and even years. Your children don't need to know every last detail of sexual function; they only need to know what they are presently asking about or are mature enough to handle. If "…the baby comes out of Mommy's tummy and joins our family…." seems to satisfy your three-year-old, leave it at that! Giving children too much information before they're ready can be just as harmful as withholding what they need to know. Don't wait to talk to your children about procreation until after they've learned about every detail in the locker room or from more experienced friends. Responding with gracious answers to their questions all throughout their childhood will help them know that you are available to openly discuss sexual issues as they grow older.

One of the easiest places to have these discussions is in the car during your daily routine. You are driving looking forward; your children are behind you. Any blushing, wincing or otherwise painful facial expressions are hidden from view as you calmly address the questions coming from the backseat. About a hundred of these comfortable and somewhat indirect talks will accomplish more than an hour spent looking across the dining room table at an uncomfortable kid who has just discovered where his Dad puts his penis.

Depending on what questions your child brings to you, you may want to defer the discussion to your partner or at least wait until they are present. Instead of brushing the question aside, simply suggest that you talk about it when Mom or Dad is available. (We found that as our children got older, they usually started approaching the parent they felt most comfortable talking to about a specific issue anyway.) Vacations are a great opportunity to have these personal conversations as everyone tends to be relaxed and there is extra time to spend together. Many of our conversations were with the whole family present; we often talked about our culture's view of sexuality, the incorrect messages being sent to youngsters and how our children could distinguish between healthy and unhealthy sexual beliefs.

You should be praying for your children's sexual protection and purity just as you do their physical health. Pray that they choose friends from healthy families who are a good influence on them. Pray that they sense such love and acceptance from family and friends that they don't go seeking it from boyfriends and girlfriends. Pray that they understand the goodness of sexuality and that shame won't play any part in their attitudes toward sex. Pray that when they have questions they'll seek you out for trustworthy answers.

In Genesis 24, Abraham sends his servant back to his family's tribe to bring back a wife for his son, Isaac. You can start praying for your child's spouse as soon as they are born! Pray for the mate of God's choosing to come into their life at the correct time; pray for strength for their parents as they raise that little boy or girl to love God and ultimately love their future husband or wife.

You should be straightforward with older children about the many consequences of sex. While avoiding unwanted pregnancy and sexually transmitted diseases isn't the *best* reason for abstaining, it's most definitely a good deterrent. Your children should understand the seriousness of all that accompanies sexual activity; not only the physical consequences, but the emotional and spiritual ones as well. Most importantly, start talking to them about how their sexuality can be used to bring glory to God. Remind them that sex is not a reward for love but a fulfillment of it. Talk about the amazing creative power of sexuality and how wonderful it is that children are the result of love between a husband and wife.

Modeling love and affection with your kids and in front of your kids lays the foundation for their sexual attitudes and expectations. It won't guarantee that your children won't dabble in sexual sin, but as they find love and acceptance within your family, the temptation to seek approval elsewhere will seem less enticing.

JUST TELL ME WHAT TO DO

❑ Are you modeling appropriate touching to your children? Is your home filled with nonsexual hugs, kisses and snuggles?

❑ Are you and your spouse modeling appropriate intimacy? Do you playfully touch each other in front of your children? Discuss ways you can give your children visible signs of your love for each other.

❑ Is there an expectation of modesty in your home, or is everyone free to walk around half-clothed? Determine to treat each person's body as precious and private. If you haven't been doing so, sit down and talk to your children about modesty. Teach every member of the family to start knocking on doors before entering a bedroom.

❑ Discuss your feelings about your gender. Do you enjoy being a man or a woman? What are your frustrations? What attitudes do you feel you're passing on to your children about their gender? What can you do to communicate that being feminine or masculine is a blessing from the Lord?

❑ Have you been using baby names for sexual anatomy? Start replacing them with correct terms.

❑ Commit to praying together as a couple for your children's sexual protection and purity. Pray for their future spouses. Pray for fulfilling, exciting sex lives for your children.

Appendix

Appendix 1

Glycemic Index

The glycemic index is defined as the blood glucose response to a 50gm available carbohydrate portion of a food expressed as a percentage of the response to the same amount of carbohydrate from a standard food, which has been either glucose or white bread. In practical terms, this means that each food has the ability to raise blood glucose to variable degrees. The greater the blood glucose level, the greater the insulin response. Thus, we want to choose food with low glycemic indices. See Table. There are many specific benefits of consuming food with low glycemic indices.

1. Blood lipids are reduced in hypertriglyceridemic patients.

2. Insulin secretion is reduced.

3. Overall blood glucose control improves in insulin-dependent and noninsulin-dependent diabetic subjects.

4. There is a reduction in abnormal blood glucose, insulin, and amino acid levels in patients with cirrhosis.

5. Urinary urea excretion is reduced, presumably by increasing nitrogen trapping by colonic bacteria.

6. Foods with low glycemic indices may enhance satiety.

7. Foods with low glycemic indices may increase athletic performance.

Glycemic Indices of Foods

FOOD	GLYCEMIC INDEX
BREADS	
Rye (crispbread)	95
Rye (whole meal)	89
Rye (whole grain, i.e. pumpernickel)	68
Wheat (white)	100
Wheat (wholemeal)	100
PASTA	
Macaroni (white, boiled 5 min)	64
Spaghetti (brown, boiled 15 min)	61
Spaghetti (white, boiled 15 min)	67
Star pasta (white, boiled 5 min)	54
CEREAL GRAINS	
Barley (pearled)	36
Buckwheat	78
Bulgur	65
Millet	103
Rice (brown)	81
Rice (instant, boiled 1 min)	65
Rice (parboiled, boiled 5 min)	54
Rice (parboiled, boiled 15 min)	68
Rice (polished, boiled 5 min)	58
Rice (polished, boiled 10–25 min)	81
Rye kernels	47
Sweet corn	80
Wheat kernels	63

FOOD	GLYCEMIC INDEX
BREAKFAST CERIALS	
"All Bran"	74
Cornflakes	121
Muesli	96
Porridge oats	89
Puffed rice	132
Puffed wheat	110
Shredded wheat	97
"Weetebix"	108
COOKIES	
Digestive	82
Oatmeal	78
Plain crackers (water biscuits)	100
"Rich Tea"	80
Shortbread cookies	88
ROOT VEGETABLES	
Potato (instant)	120
Potato (mashed)	98
Potato (new/white, boiled)	80
Potato (Russet, baked)	118
Potato (sweet)	70
Yam	74
LEGUMES	
Baked beans (canned)	70
Butter beans	46
Chickpeas (dried)	47

FOOD	GLYCEMIC INDEX
LEGUMES (Continued)	
Chick-peas (canned)	60
Frozen Peas	74
Garden peas (frozen)	65
Green peas (canned)	50
Green peas (dried)	65
Haricot beans (white, dried)	54
Kidney beans (dried)	43
Kidney beans (canned)	74
Lentils (green, dried)	36
Lentils (green, canned)	74
Lentils (red, dried)	38
Pinto beans (dried)	80
Pinto beans (canned)	38
Peanuts	15
FRUIT	
Apple	52
Apple juice	45
Banana	84
Grapes	62
Grapefruit	36
Orange	59
Orange juice	71
Peace	40
Pear	47
Plum	34
Raisins	93

FOOD	GLYCEMIC INDEX
SUGARS	
Fructose	26
Glucose	138
Honey	126
Lactose	57
Maltose	152
Sucrose	83
DAIRY PRODUCTS	
Custard	59
Ice cream	69
Skim milk	46
Whole milk	44
Yogurt	52
SNACK FOODS	
Corn chips	99
Potato Chips	77

JUST TELL ME WHAT TO DO!

❑ **One** – You can minimize sugar cravings by taking up to nine chromium tablets daily.

❑ **Two** – Keep your protein portion to three to five ounces. Large servings of protein can create sugar cravings.

❑ **Three** – Gymnema is an herb that negates the taste of "sweet."

❑ **Four** – Focus on a local source of honey as your choice of sweetener. Stevia has been used for centuries as a viable option instead of sugar.

❑ **Five** – Avoid all artificial, man-made sweeteners.

❑ **Six** – Read all labels. Evaporated can juice, raw sugar, organic crystals — are still sugar.

Appendix 2

Beet Recipes

What's great about beets –?

➢ One-half cup of cooked beets is a mere 37 calories.

➢ One-half cup has 17 percent of the Recommended Daily Intake (RDI) for folate, plus vitamin C, potassium, and iron.

➢ Beets give you the cancer-fighting antioxidant beta carotein plus 2 grams of healthy fiber.

➢ They're naturally sweet, but have only 7 grams of sugar per half-cup serving.

➢ Beets will help your body lower cholesterol up to forty percent.

Picking tips –

➢ Look for firm beets with smooth skin. Smaller ones are usually more tender than larger ones.

➢ Beets range in color from deep golden yellow to crimson to white.

➢ The lighter the color, the more mellow the flavor. The Chiggia beet is nicknamed "candy cane" because its core is striped with red and white circles.

➢ Beets are often sold with their nutritious greens attached. Avoid wilted ones and sauté them like their relative, Swiss chard.

Storing basics –

➤ Cut off the greens, leaving about one inch of stem. Place in a plastic bag and refrigerate for up to two weeks.

Cooking 101 –

➤ Keep the skins on during cooking; this helps retain moisture and nutrients. To remove the skins — and prevent staining — rub the cooked beets with a paper towel or run them under cold water while wearing rubber gloves.

➤ No time to cook? Raw beets can be peeled, grated, and tossed with a light vinaigrette for a quick, healthy salad. Spark up the flavor with grated ginger root, sesame oil, or flax oil.

Did you know...

➤ It's not an old wife's tale: Urine may turn reddish after you eat beets. This reaction, called beetura, is harmless.

RECIPES

Oven-Roasted Beets

Rub with olive oil, sprinkle with salt & pepper, and place in a roasting pan. Bake at 375°F for approximately 45 minutes, or until a knife can easily go through the center of the beet. Remove the skins, then slice and serve warm, plain or tossed with butter. Or chill the cooked beet slices and layer on top of greens. Dress with vinaigrette or flax oil, and sprinkle with toasted nuts.

Shredded Beets with Celery & Dates

Prep: about 10 minutes
Makes about 4 cups or 8 accompaniment servings

1 pound beets, peeled
3 stalks celery, thinly sliced
½ cup pitted, dried dates
3 tablespoons fresh lemon juice
Salt and coarsely ground black

Cut beets into quarters. In food processor with shredding blade attached, shred beets; transfer to a large bowl. Stir in celery, dates, lemon juice, ¼ teaspoon each salt and pepper. If not serving right away, cover and refrigerate up to 4 hours.

Each Serving: About 50 calories, 1 g protein, 13 g carbohydrate, 0 g total fat, 2 g fiber, 0 mg cholesterol, 110 mg sodium.

MAKE IT QUICK

Basil and Balsamic Beets

In 13" by 9" roasting pan, toss 2 pounds beets with 1 tablespoon olive oil. Roast in preheated 450°F oven 1 hour or until tender. Cool beets; peel and discard skins. Dice beets; toss with 2 tablespoons each chopped fresh basil and balsamic vinegar, and ¼ teaspoon Celtic Sea Salt®. Serves 4.

Each Serving: About 115 caloreis, 2 g protein, 19 g carbohydrate, 4 g total fat (0.5 g saturated), 4 g fiber, 0 mg cholesterol, 260 mg sodium.

Appendix 3

The Page Fundamental Diet Plan

One of the most common questions my patients ask me is what their diet should look like. During my post-graduate studies I spent many hours using curriculum from the International Foundation of Nutrition and Health (www.ifnh.org), which utilizes the Page Fundamental Diet Plan by Dr. Melvin Page. The plan was very logical and effective so I adapted it for use in my office.

Most people's diets seem based on about eight or ten different foods and there's little variety or excitement. It's even worse for kids who are unwilling to eat anything other than pizza, macaroni and cheese and chicken nuggets. Of course, we can't forget America's favorite vegetable: the french fry. It's a small minority who are brave enough to explore new tastes and dishes.

I'll never forget one woman who attended a workshop I gave on the drugless approach to hormone replacement therapy. At some point during the presentation I mentioned that beets can lower your cholesterol forty percent and increase liver function. Immediately following this statement I realized that this woman was staring at me rather intently. I was a bit unnerved but continued my talk. It wasn't until she approached me after the workshop that I discovered the reason for her intense gaze: this dear lady didn't know what a beet *was* or what one looked like! I was astounded but have concluded that this lack of knowledge of whole foods is quite common. So be forewarned: there are going to be foods and items mentioned in this discussion that will be foreign to you. Don't be discouraged; just be willing to try something new.

The Page Fundamental Diet Plan is designed to assist your body's ability to create and maintain "balanced body chemistry." Dr. Melvin Page's Phase 1 and Phase 2 diet is not only extremely helpful in assisting good health, but in many cases it's essential in controlling blood sugar imbalances as well as all other types of imbalanced body chemistry. Dr. Page based his diet plan on the research of Drs. Price and Pottenger, who proved the relationship of diet to both physical and emotional health. The Page plan itself was validated when blood chemistry panels of thousands of patients normalized without any other form of medical intervention. In fact, many of today's popular diets are based on Dr. Page's work. He emphasized removing refined carbohydrates (such as sugar and processed flour) and cow's milk from the diet. On the food list to follow, notice that the percentage of carbohydrates is indicated. Dr. Page also included quality carbohydrates along with quality proteins and fats.

It's been my experience that the longer patients are on this diet plan, the easier it becomes. As they develop good eating habits and their physical and emotional health levels increase, so does their resolve to make better and better choices. Old habits can be hard to break so I encourage you to make changes to your diet slowly so you don't feel overwhelmed and your body has time to adjust. There are products available that help reduce cravings.

FOODS TO CONSUME, FOODS TO AVOID

Proteins: Eat a small amount of protein at each meal. It doesn't need to be a large amount at any one time; it's best if you stick to smaller amounts (3-5 ounces of meat, fish, foul, or eggs). Both animal and vegetarian sources of protein are beneficial. Choose a variety of meat products and try to find the healthiest options available (i.e. free range, antibiotic-free and/or organic). Eggs are an excellent source of protein. Eat the whole egg as the lecithin in egg yolk is essential to lower blood fat and improve liver and brain function. The way you prepare protein to be served is critical; any time meats and vegetables are heated to over 110°F, crucial enzymes are damaged and lost. Grilled, boiled, steamed, soft boiled, or poached cooking methods are the best, and you should avoid frying foods.

Vegetables: Eat more, more, more! This is one area where almost everyone can improve their diet. Purchase a variety of vegetables but make the green leafy type your preference. This includes spinach, chard, beet greens, kale, broccoli, mustard greens, etc. As with proteins, the quality of your produce (fresh and organic when possible) and the method of preparation are critical. Raw is preferred with lightly steamed or sautéed as your second choice for all vegetables. Use primarily butter or olive oil to sauté. I also use Rice oil and coconut oil. When eating salads, avoid iceberg lettuce and opt for lettuce with a rich green color, sprouts and raw nuts. Don't make salads your only choice for veggies.

Fruits: Most people drink their fruits in the form of juices and unknowingly lose many benefits of consuming the whole fruit itself. Fruit juice is loaded with the simple sugar fructose which is made into triglycerides and ultimately stored as fat. Juice lacks the fiber found in whole fruits and sends a rapid burst of fructose into the blood stream rather than providing a slow and steady stream of energy. When you do eat fruit, eat just one kind at a time on an empty stomach. Avoid the sweetest fruits (tropical fruits) except papaya, which is very rich in digestive enzymes. Like protein and vegetables, purchase only the highest quality, fresh organic fruits as possible. I recommend you purchase fruits that are grown in your geographical region, within three hundred and fifty miles. I encourage my patients to avoid bananas, raisins, grapes, pineapple and any dried fruit. I strongly suggest pears, plums and apples.

Carbohydrates: Many people wrongly assume that carbs are carbs when in reality, carbohydrates come in three distinct types: complex (brown rice, oatmeal), simple (pears, apples) and processed (cookies, pastries). Unfortunately, all types of carbs are a no-no for patients suffering with imbalance problems. It's also a physiological fact that the more carbohydrates you eat, the more you will crave. These cravings are a symptom of an imbalance and can be used to monitor your progress. The cravings should decrease when you are effectively limiting carbs in your diet. Overall, eat vegetables as your carbohydrate choice and limit grains; even the whole grains can be trouble. When you do consume whole grains, have them in moderation and only at dinner. If you start the day with carbohydrates you're likely to crave them throughout the day, and things will just go downhill from there. Absolutely stay away from white breads, muffins, cookies, candies, crackers, pastas, white rice and most baked goods. The most sobering characteristic of processed carbo-hydrates is their connection to weight gain, elevated cholesterol and triglycerides, heart disease and cancer.

Wheat and Grains: There's been a tremendous amount of debate regarding grains. Whole unprocessed grains can be a rich source of vitamins and minerals, but with soil depletion and the genetically altered types of grain that modern agriculture has developed, it's not clear what nutrients remain in whole grain products. The two predominantly used grains in this country are genetically engineered and have five times the gluten content and only a third of the protein content of the original wheat from which they were derived. This high gluten content is to blame for many patients' allergic reactions. Scholars studying disease patterns and the decline of various civilizations have determined that many degenerative diseases developed in these populations when cultivated grains became a major part of their diets. Chemicals naturally found in certain grains, the lack of appropriate enzymes, and the carbohydrate content of grains make them a source of trouble for many individuals. I suggest minimizing grains such as wheat and barley. Unprocessed rye, rolled oats and brown rice can be considered on occasion to add more variety. You can also eat moderate amounts of Danish and German brown breads such as pumpernickel.

Sweeteners: Use only a *small* amount of raw, locally gathered honey or Stevia as a sweetener, and your diet should contain absolutely NO Nutra-Sweet®, Splenda®, corn syrup, or table sugar. Dr. Page did not allow raw sugar cane.

Fats: The bad news is that you probably don't get enough of the right fats in your diet. You should use only olive oil, cold-pressed, extra virgin, walnut, flax seed and grapeseed oils. Don't heat flax oil. These oils are actually beneficial as long as they are cold-pressed. When cooking, use only organic butter which is safe to heat. Olive oil can be heated up to 350 degrees. Avoid all hydrogenated and partially hydrogenated fats also called Trans fat, as **they are poison to your system!** Resolve to never eat margarine again. Also avoid peanut butter; eat avocados and raw nuts. I do use rice oil and coconut oil on occasion for sautéing.

If you think eating fat will make you fat, think again. When you eat fat a chemical signal is sent to your brain to slow down the movement of food out of your stomach. As a result you feel full. When you eat "fat-free" products you may tend to actually consume *more calories* than those who eat foods with unaltered fat. Those who eat the low fat, trans fat diet tend to be heavier over time. "Low-fat" usually means high sugar and high calories. In addition, fats are used not only for energy but also for building the membrane around every single cell in your body. They also play a role in the formation of hormones, and it's far worse to be hormone-depleted from a low-fat diet than it is to overeat fat. The sickest patients I treat are often those who have been on a fat-free diet for an extended period of time. Like carbohydrates, choose your fats wisely, avoiding fried and processed foods. I don't encourage the use of soy or canola oils.

Milk Products: If you knew all of the potential problems resulting from consuming *pasteurized* cow milk products (milk, certain cheeses, half and half, ice cream, cottage cheese and yogurt), you would swear off it forever. Dr. Page discovered that milk is actually more detrimental to health than sugar for many people. Man is the only mammal that continues to drink milk after being weaned off breast milk. Avoiding dairy will make it much easier for you to attain your optimum level of health and hormonal balance. *Raw* butter and Kefir (liquid yogurt), however, are excellent sources of essential nutrients and vitamins. Raw goat and sheep cheeses and milk products are great alternatives because their genetic code and fat content are apparently more similar to those of humans. You should still remain cautious with even these products.

There's been a lot of hype about using soy milk and rice milk to replace dairy. While they sound like healthy alternatives, these products are actually highly-processed foods that are primarily simple carbohydrates. You're better off avoiding them. In addition, Vitamite®, Mocha Mix®, and other dairy substitutes are highly-processed, nutrient-depleted products that should not even be considered a food.

Liquids: The best liquid you can feed your body is water, I would consume a minimum of a quart a day. I usually suggest not more than one hundred ounces, it does depend on how much you weigh. The most important life-giving substance in the body is water. The daily routine of the body depends on a turnover of about 40,000 glasses of water per day. In the process, your body loses a minimum of six glasses per day, even if you're sedentary. With movement, exercise, sugar intake, etc., you can require up to 15 glasses of water per day. Consider this — the concentration of water in your brain has been estimated to be 85 percent and the water content of your tissues (liver, kidney, muscle, heart, intestines, etc.) is 75 percent. The concentration of water outside each cell is about 94 percent. Because water by nature moves from areas of high concentration to low concentration, the water in your body continually moves across this gradient, providing hydroelectric power to your cells. This is the same electrical power generated at the Hoover Dam, functioning in miniature within you! Providing life-sustaining water to your body promotes increased energy levels, and who doesn't want more energy?!

Along with water, herbal tea is also an acceptable beverage. You should avoid all soda. Organic coffee can be added to your diet after your body is in full health, and then minimally. Fruit juices are forbidden due to their high fructose content which dumps sugar into the bloodstream. An occasional glass of eight ounces of vegetable juice that you make fresh with a meal is fine.

Alcohol should be eliminated from your diet. If you enjoy wine or beer and insist on indulging occasionally, drink it only with meals and look for organic-sourced brands. Red wine has less sugar and more of the beneficial polyphenols than white wines. Most foreign beers are actually brewed and contain far more nutrients than the pasteurized chemicals called "beer" made by the large commercial breweries in the United States. Because coffee and alcohol are diuretics and make your body lose fluids, you'll have to drink more water to compensate. Personally, I find it easier to avoid alcohol altogether.

EAT SMALLER AMOUNTS MORE FREQUENTLY

Eating smaller meals reduces the stress of digestion on your energy supply, conserving it for other routine physical tasks. Give your energy generator a chance to keep up with digestion by not overwhelming it with a large meal. The average meal time in the United States is 15 minutes; in Europe, it's 60 to 90 minutes. Little wonder Americans suffer such a high rate of digestive disorders! When digestion is impaired, yeast overgrowth, gas, inflammation and food reactions are the result.

Another reason for eating smaller meals is to prevent the ups and downs of blood sugar levels and thereby decrease sugar cravings. Just as you can overwhelm your digestive system, you can also overwhelm your body's ability to handle sugar in the blood. Since a healthy body will not allow the sugar level to get too high, insulin and other hormones are secreted to lower it. Often times the insulin response is too strong and within a short period of time it drives the blood sugar level down, resulting in powerful cravings for sugar or other carbohydrates. This leads to overeating and the cycle continues, often accompanied by depression and a lack of energy. Eating a small meal again will virtually stop this frustrating cycle.

Eating smaller meals also has advantages for your immune response to ingested food. It turns out that a small amount of food enters the blood without first going through the normal digestive pathway through the liver. As a result, this food is seen by the body not as nourishment but as a threat, stimulating an immune reaction. Normally, a small immune reaction goes unnoticed, but if a large amount of food is eaten (or if the same type of food is consumed repeatedly) the immune reaction can cause symptoms. These symptoms may include fatigue, joint aches, flu-like symptoms, headaches, etc. This reaction was named the Metabolic Rejectivity Syndrome by the late nutritional pioneer Arthur L. Kaslow, M.D. Through thousands of his patients' food diaries, he compiled a list of high-risk foods which is very similar to Dr. Page's Diet Plan.

Important Note: When in doubt, don't eat it! If a certain food isn't on the list, wait and ask your health care provider or nutritionist during your next visit. The Page Diet Plan is designed to help you reach optimal health as it has for tens of thousands of Dr. Page's patients, many of whom are in their later years without signs of degenerative diseases such as heart disease, arthritis, cancer, osteoporosis, etc. The plan is not intended to make you suffer or sacrifice. Quite the opposite is true, as you will be delighted with the physical and emotional improvements you experience from the food your body was designed to run on. What you eat and drink at the occasional party or evening out is not going to be significantly harmful to your nutritional balance in the long run, so you can enjoy occasionally straying from the diet.

Lastly, as with all things that are beneficial to your health, it may be hard to start, but the benefits greatly outweigh the struggles. The longer you use this diet, the better you'll feel and the easier it will become.

I would like to explain how to use the following food guides. The chart is based on the Glycemic Index Appendix 1, which rates how quickly glucose from each food travels in the system. Phase I focuses on items that are lower on the Glycemic Index. They will affect your blood sugar more slowly, creating a steady flow rather than spikes that create an insulin rush. The vegetables listed are loaded with minerals, especially if you focus on organic-sourced products. These particular foods will assist your body in utilizing the protein you're consuming.

When two weeks or so have passed you can then add Phase Two, which has veggies with a higher Glycemic Index number, meaning they'll stimulate a bit more insulin and get the blood glucose into the cells more quickly. Personally, I avoid the 12 – 21 percent carbs group in Phase II. I strongly encourage you to eat only the fruits included in the list. I've found that people in our society suffer from major health challenges because they focus too much on sweet fruits.

As you follow the Page Fundamental Diet Plan, remember these important points:

- ❑ Foods eaten closest to their raw state have the best digestive enzyme ability.

- ❑ Drink fluids at least one hour before or two hours after meals.

- ❑ If you insist on fluids with your meals, limit intake with to no more than four ounces.

- ❑ No processed grains, white flour, sugar or sugar substitutes.

Phase I Food Plan
For Balancing Body Chemistry
PROTEINS: MEAT — FISH — FOWL — EGGS
(See Protein Chart for Individual Portion Size)

Each of your meals must include some protein. The easiest sources are meat, fish, poultry or eggs. (Count 2 eggs as equal to 3 oz.) Vegetarians must combine proteins carefully and consistently using a different calculation. An easy way to calculate the amount of protein you need is to divide your ideal body weight by 15 to get the number of ounces of protein to be consumed per day. This is not a "high protein diet." Like many people, you already eat this much protein during a day, but you eat it mostly in one or two meals instead of spreading it out evenly over three to five meals, If you are more physically active, eat more protein.

90 lb. IBW = 6 ounces a day or 1 ¾ - 2 ounces of protein per serving.
105 lb. IBW + 7 ounces a day or 1 ¾ - 2 1/3 ounces of protein per serving.
120 lb. IBW = 8 ounces a day or 2 - 2 ¾ ounces of protein per serving.
135 lb. IBW = 9 ounces a day or 2 ½ - 3 ounces of protein per serving.
150 lb. IBW = 10 ounces a day or 3 - 3 1/3 ounces of protein per serving.
165 lb. IBW 11 ounces a day or 3 1/3 - 3 ¾ ounces of protein per serving.

IBW: Ideal body Weight

VEGETABLES: (No Limit on Serving Size)

VEGETABLES 3% or less carbs	VEGETABLES 6% or less carbs	VEGETABLES 7 – 9% carbs	OTHER FOODS In Limited Amounts
Asparagus	Bell Peppers	Acorn Squash	Butter, Raw
Bamboo Shoots	Bok Choy Stems	Artichokes	Caviar
Bean Sprouts	Chives	Avocado	Cottage Cheese, Raw
Beet Greens	Eggplant	Beets	Dressing – Oil / Cider
Bok Choy Greens	Green Beans	Brussel Sprouts	Vinegar Only
Broccoli	Green Onions	Butternut Squash	Jerky
Cabbages	Okra	Carrots	Kefir, Raw (liquid yogurt)
Cauliflower	Olives	Jicama	Milk, Raw
Celery	Pickles	Leeks	Nuts, Raw (except Peanuts)
Chards	Pimento	Onion	Oils – Vegetable, Olive (no Canola) preferably cold-pressed
Chicory	Rhubarb	Pumpkin	
Collard Greens	Sweet Potatoes	Rutabagas	
Cucumber	Tomatoes	Turnips	**BEVERAGES**
Endive	Water Chestnuts	Winter Squashes	
Escarole	Yams		Beef Tea
Garlic			Bouillon – Beef, Chicken
Kale			Herbal (Decaffeinated) Teas
Kohlrabi			Filtered or Spring Water
Lettuces			
Mushrooms			
Mustard Greens			
Parsley			
Radishes			
Raw Cob Corn			
Salad Greens			
Sauerkraut			
Spinach			
String Beans			
Summer Squashes			
Turnip Greens			
Watercress			
Yellow Squash			
Zucchini Squash			

Phase II Food Plan
For Balancing Body Chemistry

PROTEINS: MEAT — FISH — FOWL — EGGS
(See Protein Chart for Individual Portion Size)

VEGETABLES: (No Limit on Serving Size)

VEGETABLES 3% or less carbs	VEGETABLES 6% or less carbs	VEGETABLES 12 – 21% carbs	OTHER FOODS In Limited Amounts
Asparagus	Bell Peppers	*On Limited Basis*	Butter, Raw
Bamboo Shoots	Bok Choy Stems	*(Only 2-3 X/Week)*	Caviar
Bean Sprouts	Chives	Artichokes, Jerus	Cottage Cheese, Raw
Beet Greens	Eggplant	Celeriac	Dressing – Oil / Cider
Bok Choy	Green Beans	Chickpeas	Vinegar Only
Greens	Green Onions	Cooked Corn	Jerky
Broccoli	Okra	Grains, Sprouted	Kefir, Raw (liquid yogurt)
Cabbages	Olives	Horseradish	Milk, Raw
Cauliflower	Pickles	Kidney Beans	Nuts, Raw (except
Celery	Pimento	Lima Beans	Peanuts)
Chards	Rhubarb	Lentils	Oils – Vegetable, Olive
Chicory	Sweet Potatoes	Parsnips	(no Canola) preferably
Collard Greens	Tomatoes	Peas	cold-pressed
Cucumber	Water	Potatoes	
Endive	Chestnuts	Seeds, Sprouted	
Escarole	Yams	Sunflower Seeds	
Garlic			

VEGETABLES 7 – 9% carbs	FRUITS	BEVERAGES
Acorn Squash	*Limited Quantity On Limited Basis (Snacks Only)*	Beef Tea
Artichokes		Bouillon – Beef, Chicken
Avocado	Apples	Herbal (Decaffeinated)
Beets	Berries	Teas
Brussel Sprouts	Papaya	Reverse Osmosis,
Butternut	Pears	Filtered or Spring Water
Squash		Red Wine (organic
Carrots		preferred)
Jicama		
Leeks		**DESSERT**
Onion		Plain Gelatin Only
Pumpkin		
Rutabagas		
Turnips		
Winter		
Squashes		

(Kale, Kohlrabi, Lettuces, Mushrooms, Mustard Greens, Parsley, Radishes, Raw Cob Corn, Salad Greens, Sauerkraut, Spinach, String Beans, Summer Squashes, Turnip Greens, Watercress, Yellow Squash, Zucchini Squash)

Appendix 4

The Castor Oil Pack

Castor oil has been used as a natural remedy for thousands of years. While you may be familiar with its use for constipation, folk healers in this country and around the world have used castor oil for centuries to treat a wide variety of conditions. The technique is still practically unknown today. It is almost universally shunned by healthcare professions due to its profound simplicity and exotic nature, but you can't argue with the facts. I have personally seen countless numbers of patients benefit from the use of this unique oil.

And, castor oil *is* unique! Its effectiveness is probably due in part to a peculiar chemical composition. Castor oil is a triglyceride fatty acid. Almost 90 percent of its fatty acid content consists of ricinoleic acid, which isn't found in any other substance. Such a high concentration of this unusual, unsaturated fatty acid is thought to be responsible for remarkable healing abilities. Ricinoleic acid effectively prevents the growth of numerous species of viruses, bacteria, yeast and molds, explaining castor oil's success in treating such ailments as ringworm, keratoses (non-cancerous, wart-like skin growths), skin inflammation, abrasions, finger- and toenail-fungal infections, acne and chronic pruritus (itching). For topical treatment, the area involved is simply wrapped in a castor oil-soaked cloth each night. For smaller areas, an oil-soaked Band-Aid can be used. The following is a short list of some of the more common ailments that topically-applied castor oil can remedy:

- Liver spots ("Age spots")
- Skin dryness and flaking
- Wounds
- Skin cysts just below the surface
- Muscle strains
- Ringworm
- Bursitis
- Warts
- Itching
- Fungal and bacterial infections
- Abdominal stretch marks
- Ligament sprains

Castor oil can also be used as massage oil. This technique seems to be especially effective when applied along the spinal column. As the oil is rubbed into the body, the direction of the massage strokes should always follow the same path as the underlying lymphatic drainage system; start from the bottom of the spine and work up, or stroke from the extremities toward the trunk.

The most exciting way to benefit from castor oil's healing properties is to increase topical absorption through the use of packs or poultices. When the oil is absorbed through the skin, several extraordinary events take place. The lymphocyte count (white blood cells that are the "warriors" in your immune system) of the blood increases as a result of a positive influence on the thymus gland and/or lymphatic tissue. The flow of lymph increases throughout the liver and the body, speeding up the removal of toxins surrounding the cells and reducing the size of swollen lymph nodes. The end result is a general overall improvement in organ function with a lessening of fatigue and depression. Conditions related to poor drainage of the lymphatic system, toxic liver stagnation and hormonal issues all tend to respond to the use of castor oil in packs or poultices. The symptoms of these conditions include:

- ➤ Chronic fluid retention accompanied by swollen joints and pain
- ➤ Bladder and vaginal infections
- ➤ Arthritis
- ➤ Upper respiratory infections involving the sinuses, tonsils and inner ear
- ➤ Colon problems such as Crohn's Disease or colitis
- ➤ Gallbladder disease
- ➤ Liver cirrhosis, hepatitis, enlargement or congestion
- ➤ Menstrual-related congestion
- ➤ Constipation, bowel impaction or adhesions
- ➤ Swollen lymph nodes

Castor Oil Packs have been employed for health benefits since antiquity. Reportedly, they were used in ancient India, China, Persia, Egypt, Africa, Greece, Rome and in North and South America.

Necessary Articles (available at www.DruglessDoctor.com):

- ❏ Castor Oil (100% pure, cold-pressed)
- ❏ Wool Flannel (Cotton flannel should not be used)
- ❏ Heating Pad (purchase from a local store)

Procedure:

- ❏ Fold the wool flannel so that it is 3 or 4 layers thick.
- ❏ Saturate the wool flannel with castor oil.
- ❏ Place the saturated wool flannel in a baking dish and heat slowly in the oven on low heat. (Watch it carefully

so as not to burn it.) The pad should be hot but not burn the skin.

- ❑ Rub some oil onto your abdomen.

- ❑ Lay the warm wool flannel over your abdomen.

- ❑ Cover with saran wrap or plastic.

- ❑ Cover with a heating pad for one hour. It's important to keep the area as hot as possible; this is why a heating pad is recommended instead of a hot water bottle, which cools too quickly and doesn't maintain a consistent temperature.

- ❑ After an hour, remove the wool flannel and wash your skin.

- ❑ Store the wool flannel in the baking dish covered with plastic wrap or in a sealed plastic bag. (It doesn't have to be refrigerated, as castor oil is very stable and does not go rancid as other oils do.)

- ❑ If the flannel becomes discolored (other than the normal color of the oil remaining on it), it's likely from the toxins that have been drawn out of the body. I've had patients bring their cloth into the office with vibrant red, yellow, green and even purple stains. When this occurs, wash or discard the flannel.

The wool flannel may be left on for longer periods if desired. A typical treatment plan would be three consecutive days per week for as long as needed. Of course, you may use a pack more often if desired. After you experience positive results from initial treatments, once a week for the next several months is a logical protocol. The only negative side effect I've seen from the use of castor oil packs is oil-stained clothing. For this reason, I recommend you dedicate a t-shirt and pair of shorts for use at each continuing treatment.

I've recommended castor oil treatments to patients suffering from severe cervical dysplasia (abnormal tissue cells) in their uterus and/or vaginal area. After applying the packs daily for a full year, these patients have experienced the complete restoration of cellular function. In addition, I've witnessed mononucleosis respond quickly to this treatment as well as the disappearance of liver spots and cherry hemangiomas as the surface of the skin is repaired and returns to normal. Other patients using castor oil packs have seen the normalization of chronic digestive distress as a result. You should talk to your healthcare provider about this amazing natural method of promoting liver function; it's a wonderful treatment option to consider after you've modified your diet and made other necessary health changes.

Appendix 5

Marriage Assessment

We found this marriage assessment on the Discovery Channel Website — Take the time to fill it out and DISCOVER who your spouse really is… Things change — doesn't be the last person to know…

> I can name my partner's best friends.
>
> ❑ Yes
>
> ❑ no

> I can tell you what stresses my partner is currently facing.
>
> ❑ yes
>
> ❑ no

> I know the names of some of the people who have been irritating my partner lately.
>
> ❑ yes
>
> ❑ no

> I can tell you some of my partner's life dreams.
>
> ❑ yes
>
> ❑ no

> I can tell you about my partner's basic philosophy of life.
>
> ❑ yes
>
> ❑ no

➢ I can list the relatives my partner likes the least.
   ❑ yes
   ❑ no
➢ I feel that my partner knows me pretty well.
   ❑ yes
   ❑ no
➢ When we are apart, I often think fondly of my partner.
   ❑ yes
   ❑ no
➢ I often touch or kiss my partner affectionately.
   ❑ yes
   ❑ no
➢ My partner really respects me.
   ❑ yes
   ❑ no
➢ There is fire and passion in our relationship.
   ❑ yes
   ❑ no
➢ Romance is definitely still part of our relationship.
   ❑ yes
   ❑ no
➢ My partner appreciates the things I do in our relationship.
   ❑ yes
   ❑ no
➢ My partner generally likes my personality.
   ❑ yes
   ❑ no

➤ Our sex life is mostly satisfying.
   ☐ yes
   ☐ no

➤ At the end of the day my partner is glad to see me.
   ☐ yes
   ☐ no

➤ My partner is one of my best friends.
   ☐ yes
   ☐ no

➤ We just love talking to each other.
   ☐ yes
   ☐ no

➤ There is lots of give and take (both people have influence) in our discussions.
   ☐ yes
   ☐ no

➤ My partner listens respectfully, even when we disagree
   ☐ yes
   ☐ no

➤ My partner is usually a great help as a problem solver.
   ☐ yes
   ☐ no

➤ We generally mesh well on basic values and goals in life.
   ☐ yes
   ☐ no

Dr. Bob's Drugless Health Formulas

Drugless Healthcare Solutions™ has created a line of optimal health products which will be available in retail outlets, professional offices and other locations including www.druglessdoctor.com The supplements have been developed to serve as an adjunct for the recommendations that Dr. Bob has outlined in his books, CD's, DVD's and other audio applications.

Dr. Bob's Drugless Health Formulas

- ➢ Detoxification
- ➢ Whole Food Digestive Aid
- ➢ Lipid Plus – Promotes Cellular Metabolism and Liver Cleansing
- ➢ Optimal Support for Men
- ➢ Optimal Support for Women
- ➢ Adrenal Stress Formula

Closing Remarks

It is hard to say goodbye to this project that has consumed much of our lives over the past three years in the process, and past four or five in thought! It is our pleasure to bring you this book for life transformation.

Every book is only a book, with no meaning unless you take something from it. We pray you do just that and not only that but share it with others who are fulfilled, hurting, or just getting married. Our prayer is to have that touch come in at least one way to make your sexual life at least an ounce better!

Something we did recognize while we reread the book for the final time is we didn't say something more about forgiving and forgetting! That almost astonished me (Debbie) since we have had much of this our entire married lives.

This is not an easy subject for most — but a needed subject in the light of today's hurts and divisions not only in marriages but amongst family and friends.

In the word, we find Jesus had two powerful statements from the cross. We need to put more emphasis on what He was trying to teach us even with His last breaths. The first was, Father forgive them, they know not what they do. Most people don't even know that they have hurt you, even as intimate as a husband and wife relationship. Nothing is unforgivable. Nothing will tear and rip your relationship apart more that unforgiveness. Be determined to change this — turn it around and be the one that makes the most of your life.

Lastly, Jesus spoke: It is finished! As much as we herald that here with this book, know that ultimately we need to put our lives in His hands — He did it all and really knows the best. So, as we close this work — be determined to put your life in His hands.

Notes

Index

Condom use
  and unfulfilled intercourse
    104, 119 - 120
Constipation
  and painful penetration 98
Cortex 126
Cortisol 126
  anti-inflammatory response
    128
  immune system suppression
    128
  normalizing blood sugar 128
  physiology of stress 129
Created to create 85

D

Dating and/or courting 46
Depression
  factors precipitating 112
DHEA 126
Diabetes
  and sexual dysfunction 117
Diabetes-related dysfunction 103
Divorce 183
Domestic support 15
Dr. Bob's Drugless Health
  Formulas 249
Drugs and stress 172
Duloxetine (Cymbalta) 111

E

Eat smaller meals 234
Ejaculation dysfunction 103, 115 -
  116
Endocrine (or glandular) system
  27
Epididymis 170
Epinephrine 126

Erectile dysfunction 103, 105
  common dietary and
    structural factors
    precipitating 106
  common medical reasons for
    106
  due to misalignment 108
  managing 103
  medication side effects and
    109
  physiology of 107
  treating 114
Erections
  nocturnal 115
Estrogen
  in men 145
  overload 152
  saturation 174

F

Fatigue/exhaustion
  causes of 64
Fats 231
Fat-soluble vitamins 147
Feminine sexual experience 43
Fertile
  when a woman is most 78
Financial support 16
Fluorine 164
Fluoxetine (Prozac) 111
Food Plan
  Phase I 236
  Phase II 238
Foods to consume/foods to avoid
  229
Foreplay 199
French kissing 202
Fruits 229

Books by Dr. DeMaria

- ❑ Dr. Bob's Guide to Stop ADHD in 18 Days
- ❑ Dr. Bob's Trans Fat Survival Guide
- ❑ Dr. Bob's Guide to Optimal Health
- ❑ Dr. Bob's Drugless Guide to Detoxification
- ❑ Dr. Bob's Drugless Guide to Longevity
- ❑ Dr. Bob's Drugless Guide to Balancing Female Hormones

Order the books wholesale or retail at:
www.druglessdoctor.com

Products and Services available by Dr. DeMaria

- ❑ Visit our web site and sign up for the weekly e-tips
- ❑ Link on to the secure Maestro Symptom Survey Link and receive a computerized report with nutritional recommendations

www.druglessdoctor.com

Special Appearances, Radio and TV Events

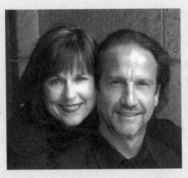

Dr. Bob and Debbie are available on a limited basis to speak at your next Event or Convention. Their energetic speaking style will inspire, educate and motivate your team to greater levels of health and personal confidence. The DeMarias' enthusiasm for life is **contagious!**

To schedule or inquire please call:

1.888.922.5672

or email: druglesscare@aol.com